THE ESSENCE OF BACH FLOWERS

*Traditional and Transpersonal
Use and Practice*

THE ESSENCE OF BACH FLOWERS

*Traditional and Transpersonal
Use and Practice*

by
Rachelle Hasnas, MSW
Certified Bach Flower Practitioner

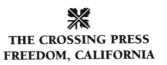

**THE CROSSING PRESS
FREEDOM, CALIFORNIA**

Permissions

Grateful acknowledgment is made to the following for permission to reprint from:

Anatomy of the Spirit, by Caroline Myss, copyright 1996. Reprinted by permission of Harmony Books.

The Bach Flower Remedies, by Dr. Bach and Dr. Wheeler, copyright 1979 by the Edward Bach Healing Centre. Reprinted by permission of Keats Publishing, Inc., in arrangement with the C. W. Daniel Publishing Company Ltd.

The Edgar Cayce Readings: #1967-1, 262-83, and 4016-1. Reprinted by permission of The Edgar Cayce Foundation.

Vibrational Medicine, by Dr. Richard Gerber, copyright 1988. Quoted by permission of Bear & Company.

Wheels of Life, by Anodea Judith, copyright 1987. Reprinted by permission of Llewellyn Publications.

Dr. Edward Bach, Bach Flower Remedies, Bach Flower Essences, and Rescue Remedy are trademarks of Bach Flower Remedies, Ltd., Oxfordshire, England.

The information contained in this book is not meant to give specific recommendations for the treatment of any disease or symptoms of disease—mental or physical. It has been written as a review of the Bach Flower Essences, an alternative therapy that may be used as a *complementary approach* in conjunction with traditional medical treatments. This book is not meant to replace good medical diagnosis and treatment. It is suggested that the reader seek the advice of a trained health-care practitioner whenever necessary.

Library of Congress Cataloging-in-Publication Data

Hasnas, Rachelle.
    Essence of Bach flowers : traditional and transpersonal use and
practice / by Rachelle Hasnas.
        p. cm.
    Includes bibliographical references and index.
    ISBN 0-89594-969-5
    1. Flowers—Therapeutic use. 2. Homeopathy—Materia medica and
therapeutics I. Title.
RX615.F55H367 1999
615'.321—dc21   98-53511
                                                      CIP

This book is dedicated to the Healer Within—
The Spirit of Life in each of us.
That Its presence be made conscious in you—
To ever guide you on your journey to wholeness.

Acknowledgments

First and foremost, I honor and thank the Creator of All That Is, our Mother/Father God, for guiding and supporting me in bringing this book into manifestation. I also am grateful beyond words to Dr. Edward Bach, whose spirit fills these pages. His work has been an inspiration and catalyst for my personal healing as it has been and will continue to be for so many others.

I also extend very special thanks to my precious son Daniel for allowing me the space to write without interruption and making sure I didn't forget to eat and sleep; to my beloved son Joshua, for inspiring me to go on and write a bigger book; and to a very dear and special friend, Ann Carricato. Her encouragement and support of the artist within me has been uplifting and unfailing beyond measure.

And most significantly, for believing in my work with the publication of The Essence of Bach Flowers, I deeply thank Elaine Goldman Gill, the publisher of The Crossing Press, and Jill Schettler, the acquisitions editor. Heart-felt appreciation also goes to my editor, David McIrvine, for his many hours of dedication in bringing my manuscript into its final form. He clarified and articulated facts without changing my thinking or the general flow of my words. His skill is a true art. And my final, and most special, thank you is saved for Cyndi Barnes—an angel in disguise! I've been truly blessed by her support of my work.

—Rachelle Hasnas

Contents

The cure of the part should not be attempted without treatment of the whole. No attempt should be made to cure the body without the soul, and, if the head and body are to be healthy, you must begin by curing the mind...For this is the great error of our day in the treatment of the human body, that physicians first separate the soul from the body.

—Plato, *The Republic*

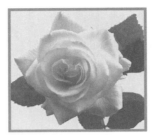

Introduction

I welcome you with great joy and hope in what I trust will be a journey of self-empowerment...a journey of taking your personal power back in regard to healing—power that you will know lies within you. Consciousness is the first step: doing something about it then becomes your choice.

My purpose in writing this book is to bring new understanding to the way we view health and what healing is really about. Perhaps you are already generally aware of this information, yet have not made the effort to bring it into your life actively. If so, then I trust that what you read will act as a reminder for you, and will inspire you to take another look at these concepts.

Although this book focuses on the Bach Flower Essences themselves, I wish to emphasize Dr. Bach's insights into the basis of health. His holistic self-healing system of flower essences is only one of the many existing methods that facilitate well-being. The underlying view of health versus disease that Dr. Bach has brought to us is the door in symbolic terms, and his flower essences but one of numerous keys that allow us access to our true source of healing.

It is not the medicine we ingest or medical procedure (surgery, etc.) we undergo that heals us. These merely enhance the natural healing ability that we all possess deep within ourselves. We need to understand and embrace this concept for our highest good: doing so we enter upon a path that will empower us as never before.

If you are reading this book it is an indication that you are ready to view health in a new light, that you are taking responsibility for your health in a new way—a holistic way. Wholism must be recognized and implemented in our lives on many levels. We have been fragmented for too long in our materialistic, mechanistic, scientific worldview that has been the determining factor of our reality.

It is now time to put the pieces back together and acknowledge that we are multidimensional beings, a complex of body, mind, and spirit intertwined. With this recognition we reclaim our divine heritage as children of God. One of the purposes in our being here on planet Earth is to remember that we are spiritual beings first and foremost. Once we incarnated, most of us forgot who we are, and the veil of separation came between us and our Source. This separation is truly an illusion, for our spiritual connection, though forgotten, can never be broken.

As the new millennium approaches, a shift in consciousness appears to be at hand—a paradigm shift in our worldview. The transpersonal aspect of self is being resurrected. The term "transpersonal" can be defined as a sense of identity of self that extends beyond the individual or the personal. The transpersonal experience encompasses wider facets of humankind, life, and the psyche, and reaches out to include the cosmos itself.

This concept comprises both the inner and outer worlds, our introspective and our sensory experiences, within one reality, neither having more importance than the other. In fact, we have to embrace both in order for any expansion of consciousness to take place. Thus, opening to the transpersonal may been seen as a journey towards greater self-awareness, healing, and empowerment. We are awakening to the spirit within and remembering our very soul.

With this concept as my inspiration, I have taken the transpersonal into consideration in the writing of this book, knowing the treatment of more than just the physical is presently needed in our approach to healing. As many of us, separately and collectively, are now becoming conscious of this transpersonal element in our lives, it seems to be the perfect time to present information along these lines. And I have endeavored to execute this with *The Essence of Bach Flowers*.

Part One is devoted to traditional Bach Flower Essence use and practice. You are given the basics and also other pertinent information about this extraordinary self-help healing system. In Part Two, your vision is expanded beyond the physical. Here, the transpersonal is explored by

- Incorporating the use and practice of Dr. Bach's method with affirmations to harness the power of your mind (for greater flower essence efficacy)
- Complementing Bach Flower Essence selection with astrological insight into your Personality Type Essence, Life Issues, and Transits (for personal growth)
- Regaining your personal power with the unblocking of the chakras that Bach Flower Essences afford (for emotional healing on all levels)
- Discovering the transcendent through your discipline and practice of meditation.

With this unique approach to Dr. Bach's work, I have attempted to present a broader perspective on flower essences and their use. This view encompasses both the traditional and the transpersonal, as so many of us are beginning to sense that we are more than physical beings and that life has a deeper meaning and purpose than we ever imagined.

We are told by Dr. Bach that "Life does not demand of us unthinkable sacrifice; it asks us to travel its journey with joy in our heart and to be a blessing to those around us, so that we leave this world just a trifle better for our visit, then we have done our work."

To this end I offer *The Essence of Bach Flowers* so that your journey may be more joyful and fulfilling and your presence a blessing to others, and so that, when you leave this world, it has been graced by your visit...

Part One

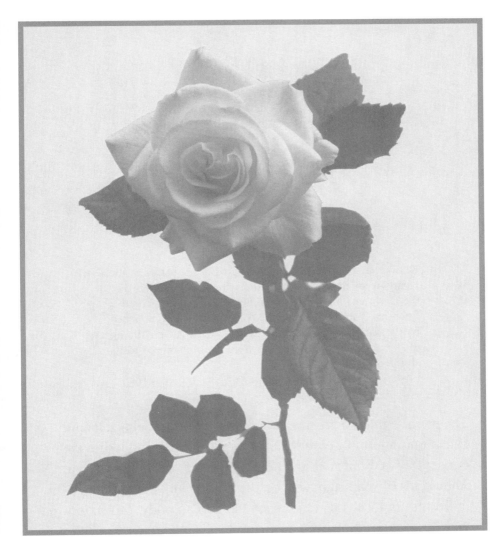

T**RADITIONAL** U**SE** & P**RACTICE**

1.

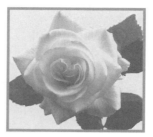

Vibrational Medicine

Know that all strength, all healing of every nature is the changing of the vibrations from within—the attuning of the Divine within the living tissue of the body to Creative Energies. This alone is healing. Whether it is accomplished by the use of drugs, the knife or whatnot, it is the attuning of the atomic structure of the living cellular force to its spiritual heritage.

—*Edgar Cayce,* Reading 1967-1

The premise that we are much more than physical beings, that in fact at our innermost core we are energetic beings, underlies the concept of vibrational medicine. This is not a new idea. Thousands of years ago, well before the advent of modern medicine and its mechanistic view of the human body, this axiom was honored and utilized in many traditions throughout the world. Shamans, healers, and adepts in the mystery schools of ancient times, as well as those with intuitive abilities, have been aware of the subtle energetic field that permeates the physical body. Their healing practices were directed towards this subtle energy field where mind, body, and spirit merged.

It was also accepted long ago that disease did not begin on the material plane, but within the layers of this subtle energy field. It was understood that distress or disharmony initially ingrained itself within these subtle layers—on the emotional and mental levels. Once established here, the discord infiltrated the body's energetic system as a whole. Should this disequilibrium continue without the restoration of harmony, the physical body became vulnerable to the inception of disease. Thus, illness of the body was seen as the final outcome of an imbalance that was not physical.

Humanity has lost touch with this ancient wisdom. For centuries we have been indoctrinated with a medical model that sees the body as a machine. In the last few decades the old paradigm has begun to be seriously challenged with the advent of mind-body medicine. That our thoughts and feelings play a significant part in determining our state of health is once again acknowledged.

Traditional Western medicine is beginning to recognize that when we are emotionally upset or mentally distressed, our health suffers. The old model can't explain this. Medical scientists are now discovering that there are other factors beyond the physical that must also be addressed.

To this end, a relatively new branch of medicine, Psycho-neuroimmunology (PNI), has begun to examine the mind-body connection and its relationship to disease. It is now accepted that stress plays a major role in the manifestation of disease. This mind-body link has been scientifically proven in research laboratories nationwide.

PNI has now established that during stressful situations and negative emotional states, the brain produces neurotransmitters that are toxic to the body's immune system. Conversely, during pleasurable situations and positive emotional states, the brain also produces neurotransmitters which enhance the body's immune system. Treating the whole person (body, mind, and spirit) is now gaining acceptance within the medical establishment.

With the medical profession's recognition that stress-producing thoughts and emotions have a negative effect upon our physical well-being, vibrational medicine has come upon the scene.

Dr. Larry Dossey applauded vibrational medicine as an idea whose time has come, and commented at the beginning of Dr. Richard Gerber's revolutionary book *Vibrational Medicine*, "Anyone who is aware of the recent trends in medicine will realize that the modern physician—like the physicists before them—have begun to deal with finer and finer forms of energy both in the diagnosis and treatment of human illness. This trend can only continue. It is sure to bring with it the recognition of increasingly subtle expressions of our minds and bodies, which will require correspondingly subtler approaches in therapy."

Dr. Gerber has brought us a revolutionary new model of healing, which recognizes that consciousness and body merge; that in fact we are multidimensional beings in whom spirit gives life to the physical. He asks us to no longer picture ourselves merely as mechanical beings. He brings us an alternative view on healing. In the medicine of the future, the treatment of both mind and spirit will become crucial factors. If not, Gerber maintains, medical intervention will continue to fall short, because it leaves out the most fundamental quality of human existence—the spiritual dimension. The element of spirit—along with oxygen, glucose, and other chemical nutrients—nourishes our physical form with higher vibrational energies; spirit is at the very heart of sustaining life itself.

Vibrational medicine is based upon the Einsteinian paradigm. Through his famous equation, $E = mc^2$, Albert Einstein demonstrated to the world that matter and energy are dual expressions of the nature of the universe. We are all composed of this primal energy or vibration. The Einsteinian paradigm, as applied to vibrational medicine, envisions human beings as networks of complex energy fields that mesh within the physical/cellular systems. We are healthy as long as balance is maintained on all levels. If this equilibrium is disrupted at higher levels, the body will reflect this disharmony through the development of disease.

Vibrational medicine restores order from a higher level of functioning, by rebalancing the energy fields that help to regulate the physical system. Instead of using conventional drugs and surgical approaches, vibrational medicine treats people with pure energy. It uses "frequency specific" forms of energy to positively affect the unbalanced energetic systems that have manifested disease.

Dr. Gerber explains, "This theoretical perspective is based upon the understanding that the molecular arrangement of the physical body is actually a complex network of interwoven energy fields. The energetic network, which represents the physical/cellular framework, is organized and nourished by 'subtle' energetic systems which coordinate the life-force with the body. There is a hierarchy of subtle energetic systems that coordinate electro-physiologic, hormonal function, as well as cellular structure within the physical body. It is primarily from these subtle levels that health and illness originate. These unique energy systems are powerfully affected by our emotions and level of spiritual balance as well as by nutritional and environmental factors. These subtle energies influence cellular patterns of growth in both positive and negative directions."

By working with the energetic patterns that influence the physical expression of life, vibrational medicine strives to heal illness, and bring consciousness to a higher level. Dr. Gerber predicts that we will eventually discover that consciousness itself is an energy, and that it is intimately related to the cellular expression of our physical body. Thus, consciousness participates in the unending creation of either health or illness.

This is a profound concept, reflecting the awesome (and mostly unconscious) power of the mind and its effect on the body. As we move into the new millennium, vibrational medicine's revolutionary approach to the treatment of disease will surely be recognized as a beacon of light by physicians. It may conceivably show doctors why some individuals remain healthy while others are continually in a state of disease.

I found it extraordinary to discover that over half a century ago, renowned English physician, bacteriologist, and medical researcher, Dr. Edward Bach, was also aware of these modern concepts. This was before the advent of such concepts as the mind-body link or vibrational medicine. He also recognized that disease was an outgrowth of the dysfunctional vibrational patterns within the body's subtle energetic systems.

Dr. Bach was truly a pioneer and a man well ahead of his time, with an extraordinary and unparalleled understanding and insight into the healing process. Compelled by a profound desire to find a fresh approach to this subtle energetic system, Dr. Bach searched for a new method of healing, a holistic *method*, that treated the whole person. He is now considered "the Father of Vibrational Medicine."

Dr. Bach's new system was based on his perception that disease was a reflection of misalignment between the personality and the soul. He believed that materialism ignored the factor above the physical plane that provided protection or rendered a person susceptible to disease. He cited fear as one example, convinced that it caused disharmony in our physical and magnetic bodies and opened the way for the invasion of illness through its depressing effect on our mentality.

For Dr. Bach, the true cause of disease was located in the personality, where emotional and mental disharmony were the precursors. It was his contention that the future of healing would advance beyond primarily physical methods of treating the body to spiritual and mental healing. By bringing harmony between the soul and personality, the initial cause of disease would be eradicated. Physical means would still be used, but only to complete the cure of the body when necessary.

Dr. Bach's development of his flower remedies, currently known around the world as the Bach Flower Essences, is now viewed as the origin of vibrational medicines. These subtle vibrational energies contained within the flower essences catalyze the realignment of an individual's emotional patterns of dysfunction. This reinstates the proper vibrational frequencies necessary for the restoration of health and well-being.

Dr. Bach's unorthodox, holistic approach to the treatment of disease with his new system of healing was not accepted by the medical profession during his life. Now, the medical paradigm is abandoning the old mechanistic model that views the body as a machine. It begins to recognize what the New Age rediscovered—that we are, indeed, multidimensional beings. The Bach Flower Essences are accordingly being recognized as a viable intervention in the treatment of disease.

Both Dr. Bach and Dr. Gerber have brought to us a new scientific paradigm which strongly supports what certain healers and visionaries have known for thousands of years. This may enable us to shift from the fragmented, mechanistic understanding of health to the unbroken wholeness of the Einsteinian worldview that embraces the concept of matter as a form of energy.

The next chapter will explore the events that prompted Dr. Bach's withdrawal from traditional medicine and led to his search for a new approach to healing. It will also explain Dr. Bach's underlying philosophy of health, which prompted the ensuing development of the Bach Flower Essences.

2.

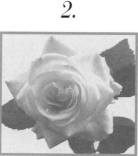

Dr. Bach's Approach to Healing

Thus we see that our conquest of disease will mainly depend on the following: firstly, the realization of the Divinity within our nature and our consequent power to overcome all that is wrong; secondly, the disharmony between the personality and the Soul; thirdly, our willingness and ability to discover the fault which is causing such a conflict; and fourthly, the removal of any such fault by developing the opposing virtue.

—*Edward Bach,* The Twelve Healers

Dr. Bach was a healer in the deepest sense of the word. Even as a young boy he felt a profound desire to heal and help humanity. In 1906, at the age of twenty, this heartfelt calling eventually led to his study of medicine. From that moment on, Dr. Bach's enthusiasm and intense desire to heal totally filled his life—with room for little else.

During his early years as a physician, it became apparent to him that the real study of pathology was in the scrutiny of the patient and her personality. He saw that the same procedure did not always cure the same disease in all patients. With this new awareness he began to question the current medical practice of standard treatments for specific diseases. Eventually, he began to also notice that patients with a similar personality would often respond to the same treatment regardless of their particular disease. Those individuals with different personalities needed other medical attention, although they experienced the same disease.

In this way Dr. Bach came to understand that it was the personality of an individual that was more important than the body in regard to the treatment of disease. This remarkable insight— treat the individual, not the disease—became the cornerstone of the new system of medicine that he would develop some twenty years later.

Bach was a brilliant physician, steeped in the science of medicine. Yet, he was also a man of profound sensitivity and intuition. These qualities led him to break away from traditional medicine. After an illness that almost took his life, Bach knew he had to leave London. Because he was extremely sensitive, the noise and crowds of the busy city were taking their toll on his health. Within a short time, he gave up his lucrative medical practice and moved to the English countryside, where he intuitively felt he would find what he sought. Thus, he began his search among the flowers and trees of the field, returning to nature for the new form of healing he longed to find.

Dr. Bach was so finely tuned that he could actually sense the subtle energies within the morning dew on the flowers as he touched them. In this manner he could also discern their potential therapeutic effects. His intuition had served him well. In the countryside, he would eventually find the thirty-eight flower essences that would comprise the holistic system of healing he had envisioned.

What initially catalyzed his search for a new way of healing was his disenchantment with traditional medical treatment. Through his personal observations of his patients over many years, he was convinced that the medicine of his day was merely treating the symptoms of disease, without touching the root cause. Bach was convinced that if the cause was not addressed, no lasting cure would be possible. He believed that the main reason for the failure of modern medicine was that it dealt with results, and not with causes.

It was his unequivocal belief that one's negative states of mind and emotions lay at the very heart of the manifestation of an illness. Our state of health was directly linked to our state of mind. In his quest for other medical treatment that would address this connection, the door to homeopathy was opened to him. Bach had a strong affinity for the ideas of homeopathic practice. These ideas led him toward the new form of healing he had sought for so long.

Dr. Bach's search for a new model of healing was nourished by his underlying profound spiritual philosophy, which directly informed his theory of the true cause of disease. In *Heal Thyself*, Dr. Bach writes, "It cannot be too firmly realized that every Soul in incarnation is down here for the specific purpose of gaining experience and understanding and perfecting his personality towards those ideals laid down by the Soul. Let everyone remember that his Soul has laid down for him a particular work, and that unless he does this work, though perhaps not consciously, he will inevitably raise a conflict between his Soul and personality which of necessity reacts in the form of physical disorders..."

It would seem from Dr. Bach's comments that he was well versed in reincarnation theory in which we, as souls, incarnate for a specific mission or purpose. When the personality becomes misaligned with the purpose of the soul, a disharmony on an energetic level is created, with the eventual manifestation of disease if harmony is not re-established. Dr. Bach developed his flower essences to restore this balance and harmony between the personality and the soul.

Bach Flower Essences do *not* treat any disease or symptoms of disease. There are no Bach Flowers that treat cancer or diabetes or any other physical illness. What they *do* treat are the underlying negative emotional and mental states that are the very cause of disease. Thus, we choose the flower essences that are appropriate for treating our negative emotions and states of mind, and our personality faults that cause disharmony and distress. These imbalances indicate which particular flower essence, or essences, will best address and treat our discomfort.

In our use of flower essences it is imperative that we are in touch with what is going on within. What is it that is bringing unhappiness and distress (dis-ease) to us? Are we bitter or resentful? In denial or repressing our feelings? Are we lacking self-worth or feeling hopeless, suspicious, or jealous? Do we live in fear? Are we uncertain of our path in life? Do we display intolerance towards others? These are just a few of the many possible negative emotions, states of mind, and personality faults that promote illness for us if they are not remedied.

The Bach Flower Essences facilitate the release and healing of these and any other negative feelings and states of mind that exist. In all, there are thirty-eight different flower essences, as well as one very special combination formula that Dr. Bach developed—the Rescue Remedy. Rescue is comprised of five of the thirty-eight essences. When he completed his self-help healing system, Dr. Bach felt that these thirty-nine essences addressed all known negative states of mind.

Surprisingly, Dr. Bach considered disease itself to be beneficial. Illness is a wake-up call from our soul, which reminds us that we are out of alignment with our life's purpose. Disease only comes to us as a signal to nudge us back on track, to be true to ourselves and the higher purpose for which we were born. It is of no importance how insignificant or grand our life may be in the eyes of the world. It isn't what we do, but the love and sense of peace and harmony we feel for what we are doing that matters. It is our intention that matters.

Dr. Bach had come to fully understand the importance of *treating the whole person*—body, mind, and spirit. His development of the flower essences was directly related to this concept, which is clearly indicated in *Heal Thyself*: "From time immemorial it has been known that Providential Means have placed in nature the prevention and cure of disease, by means of divinely enriched herbs and plants and trees. They have been given the power to heal all types of illness and suffering. In treating cases with these remedies no notice is taken of the nature of the disease. The individual is treated, and as he becomes well the disease goes, having been cast off by the increase of health. The mind, being the most delicate and sensitive part of the body, shows the onset and course of the disease much more definitely than the body, so that the outlook of mind is chosen as the guide as to which remedy or remedies is necessary..."

Dr. Bach also believed that the dawn of a new and better model of healing would soon arrive. He wrote, "A hundred years ago the Homeopathy of Hahnemann was as the first streak of morning light after a long night of darkness, and it may play a big part in the medicine of the future..." Let us hope so.

Dr. Bach was also a firm believer in the practice of daily meditation, in taking the time to ponder and explore one's innermost self. He felt this was one very helpful way of connecting with the higher self or soul. Through the practice of meditation, we are given a simple way to open to, and receive, guidance from our higher self. Through meditation our spiritual evolution is also facilitated by the expansion of our consciousness, thus bringing us a deeper alignment with our soul and its purpose.

Dr. Bach believed that we all have the inherent ability to create peace, health, and fulfillment in our lives. In fact, this is our divine right and heritage. In order that we understand the true nature of disease, Bach puts forth certain fundamental truths or principles in *Heal Thyself.*

First and foremost, Dr. Bach states that we each have a soul which is our true self. We are divine beings, the sons and daughters of the Creator of all things. Our body is but the earthly temple of that soul, and it is only an infinitesimal reflection.

Second, we as souls, have incarnated to gain all the knowledge and experience which can be obtained by earthly life. We are meant to develop virtues which we may lack and eradicate whatever personality flaws we may possess, as we advance towards the perfection of our true natures. The soul knows the perfect situations and circumstances we need to enable us to do this. Where we are in life is no accident.

Third, our life on earth is only a moment in the course of our evolution. Our souls are immortal, and our bodies are merely temporary, given to us as instruments for the work we've come to do.

His fourth principle cites the importance of the alignment between soul and personality for the maintenance of joy, peace, and health. When conflict arises, either by our own desires and faults, or created by the influence of others, we open ourselves to the causes of disease.

Dr. Bach's final principle emphasizes the understanding of the unity of all things and the fact that the Creator of all things is Love. Everything of which we are conscious, from the farthest galaxy to the lowest form of life, is a manifestation of that Love. Therefore, any action taken against ourselves, or against another, affects the whole. We go against this unity with two great possible fundamental errors: dissociation between our souls and personalities, and any cruelty or wrong done to another. And by these very actions we bring discord upon ourselves, thereby opening the door to disease.

Dr. Bach then stresses, "That by its very principles and in its very essence, disease is both preventable and curable, and it is the work of spiritual healers and physicians to give, in addition to material remedies, the knowledge to the suffering of the error of their lives, and of the manner in which these errors can be eradicated, and so to lead the sick back to health and joy."

This is becoming evident today, especially in the treatment of cancer. Medical researchers, as well as physicians, are now noticing that those patients who remain in remission have not only made changes in lifestyle (diet, exercise, etc.), but have made a shift in consciousness. It appears that these individuals came to a new understanding regarding their lives, recognizing that new ways of thinking and being were also essential. Yes, the body was treated for the disease, but, unless emotional, mental, and personality shifts took place, the disease would return.

Dr. Bach had found what he had been looking for with the development of his flower essences, fulfilling his particular mission in life. And in his doing so it has become a blessing and gift to the world. By his taking on this great service for humankind, we have been given a most remarkable healing modality and precursor to the medicine of the future. Bach Flower Essences are so safe and gentle in their effect, they can be used even during pregnancy. They are non-addictive, do not produce side effects, and there is no danger of overdosing. They can be safely taken while using other medication without hampering the effects of either. And flower essences have an indefinite shelf-life, if kept in a dark, cool place.

Dr. Bach made his system of flower essences a simple one, so that even people without medical knowledge could benefit from it. He saw that an individual only needed to be in touch with the negative states of mind, emotions, or character traits that were causing distress. Once these were understood, it was easy to select the flower essences that were needed. Dr. Bach stated that using his flower essences should be this simple: When a person is hungry, she goes to the garden and picks some lettuce; when a person is feeling fear, she takes a dose of Mimulus (the flower essence that addresses a fearful state of mind).

The bottle of concentrate contains pure spring water, brandy as a preservative, and the particular essence or vibration of one of the specific thirty-eight flowers that facilitates the release of a certain negative emotion or state of mind. The flower essences themselves are obtained by one of two methods—the sun method or by boiling—as originally prepared by Dr. Bach.

SUN METHOD OF POTENTIZATION

Several blossoms of the particular flower essence that is being prepared are placed in glass bowls of spring water, and then placed outside in the sun for approximately three to four hours.

BOILING METHOD OF POTENTIZATION

For the flowers he chose that bloomed early in the spring, Dr. Bach determined that the sun was not hot enough to effectively potentize the water. Thus, he boiled these blossoms in spring water for approximately thirty minutes.

In both methods, the water is impregnated with the therapeutic vibration contained in the specific flower. The mother tincture is then made by straining all physical components of the flowers from the original solution, and then adding an equal amount of brandy as a preservative.

Again, the selection of a particular flower essence is chosen according to one's negative state of mind, emotions, and personality. As an example, for an individual who is suffering from low self-esteem, the flower essence that relates to this indication would be Larch. The healing energy or vibration contained in Larch is that of *Confidence*. The energetic system of the person needing this flower essence would be flooded by the vibration of confidence, bringing the eventual release of the negative state of inferiority and lack of self-worth. As another example, for an individual with a personality prone to impatience, a trait known to cause a great deal of stress and tension, the flower essence Impatiens is indicated. Its vibration of *Patience* would then restore harmony to this individual's system.

Actually, according to Dr. Bach, we each have within us all the positive virtues since we're are all spiritual beings, and these assist us in remaining healthy when they are active. Regrettably, these virtues are often covered or blocked by our negative emotions and states of mind. The flower essences are similar to catalysts in that they uncover or unblock these hidden virtues (healing life energy). Once this is freed and active, our well-being is again promoted with the mobilization of the true healing process—that which starts from within.

I, along with other practitioners, have found that, with the use of Bach Flower Essences, success has been achieved in relieving long-standing patterns of emotional anxiety as well as personality dysfunction.

Let us now take an in-depth look at these incredible gifts of nature as we move on to the next chapter, and what may become for you a remarkable support system for your healing process.

3.

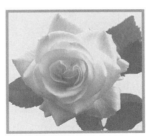

A Review of the "39 Healers"

From time immemorial it has been known that Providential Means have placed in Nature the prevention and cure of disease, by means of divinely enriched herbs and plants and trees. The remedies of Nature given (in this book) have proved that they are blest above others in their work of mercy; and they have been given the power to heal all types of illness and suffering.

—*Edward Bach,* The Twelve Healers

The thirty-nine healers include Dr. Bach's thirty-eight individual flower essences, and his only composite remedy—Rescue Remedy. Rescue contains five of the thirty-eight essences, and plays a vital role in the Bach Flower repertoire.

We will now explore the indications that correlate to each of the Bach Flowers and your possible need for those that relate to any of your negative states of mind, emotions, and personality traits. Keep pen and paper handy to note those that "speak to you"—those you recognize as causes of stress personally, in relationships, or in life situations. Once you've concluded your study of all thirty-nine flower essences, use your notes to help determine which essences you need.

As you go on to work with the flower essences, you will realize that this is a process of self-discovery. You will soon become aware of any personality traits, beliefs, and emotions that may be holding you back from living a richer and more fulfilling life. You will also find out any personal issues that prevent you from experiencing more joy and peace. The keys to your personal growth and emotional healing are honesty and humility. I deeply urge you to remember and honor this in achieving the greatest success in your personal healing process.

It is important that you choose the essences according to their negative indications only, not for the positive virtues that they possess. This is extremely important to remember for maximum benefit in flower essence practice and use. Dr. Bach created his system to facilitate healing when you choose an essence for the corresponding imbalanced states of mind, emotions, and personality faults that cause you distress. The positive virtue contained in any of the flower essences then re-establishes balance and harmony for that particular negative state or issue. They basically work as an "antidote," as they counteract and release the negative energy you are holding.

With the understanding of how to determine your selections, let us begin our exploration of the "39 Healers." We will examine them within the seven categories that were originally presented by Dr. Bach:

1. Essences for Fear
2. Essences for Uncertainty
3. Essences for Insufficient Interest in Present Circumstances
4. Essences for Loneliness
5. Essences for Oversensitivity to Influences and Ideas
6. Essences for Despondency or Despair
7. Essences for Over-care for Welfare of Others

ESSENCES FOR FEAR

Rock Rose

Indication: Panic and Terror

This flower essence was initially termed "the Rescue Remedy" by Dr. Bach (not to be confused with the composite formula, Rescue Remedy. Rock Rose, however, is one of the five essences contained in Rescue). It is indicated for any emergency situation when panic and terror arise. Rock Rose is excellent after a great fright. We've all seen movies in which a particular character becomes hysterical and someone slaps him in the face. Usually, the hysterical character then remarks, "Thanks, I needed that!" This situation perfectly depicts the Rock Rose state.

Many times, we experience the Rock Rose state during and after a nightmare, with feelings of hysteria, panic, and terror rising up. The emotional climate during the stock market crash of 1929 likely produced this state in many individuals.

The positive vibration of Rock Rose is *Steadfastness*. Rock Rose has bright yellow flowers, blooming from late May through August.

Mimulus

Indication: Fear from a Known Cause

Are you generally a fearful individual, timid and shy in manner? Does your fearful nature hold you back from maximum experience of life? If so, Mimulus would be indicated for you. It is also the flower essence for fear of *known* things, fears that you can verbalize and put your finger on. These include fear of illness, fear of death, fear of rejection, fear of intimacy, fear of poverty, fear of public speaking, fear of success, fear of heights, fear of water, fear of snakes, fear of flying, and other fears too numerous to cite.

Phobias, though irrational, are also known fears. Again, Mimulus would be indicated. Most of us remember the Cowardly Lion in *The Wizard of Oz*. This character seemed always in a state of fear and longed for courage above all. This is a vivid depiction of the Mimulus state.

The positive vibration of Mimulus is *Courage*. Mimulus has bright yellow flowers with a few red spots on the lower lip, blooming from June through August.

Cherry Plum
Indication: Fear of Loss of Control
Are there times when you feel out of control? That you may do something harmful to yourself, or to another? Do you indulge in temper tantrums, and recognize that you have a temper that controls you? Are you prone to outbursts? Do you take risks that are physically dangerous, enjoying the sense of danger? Are you out of control with credit card use, gambling, or use of drugs and alcohol? Do you actually hit others, or feel you might do so one day? These are all examples of the negative Cherry Plum state.

In any situation where you feel you're losing control over any action you take, or are prone to impulsive acts that are detrimental to your well-being, Cherry Plum is indicated. Cherry Plum is one of the flower essences that is very helpful with suicidal thinking, as well as with obsessive-compulsive behavior. The out-of-balance Cherry Plum state is obvious in rock stars who have overdosed on drugs.

The positive vibration of Cherry Plum is *Composure*. The cherry plum tree's flower is pure white and blooms from late February to early April.

Aspen
Indication: Foreboding, Apprehension
With Aspen we are looking at *unknown fear* and our inability to put our finger on what we are afraid of. There is a sense of

apprehension and diffuse anxiety in this state that produces a fear of the unknown. Individuals who suffer from states of anxiety, bringing on panic attacks, do extremely well with Aspen. It is also suggested for those suffering from phobias to be used in conjunction with Mimulus. Aspen also reduces feelings of foreboding—that "creepy crawly" sensation that can come upon us for no apparent reason.

This essence is also indicated for individuals who are overly superstitious, as well as those who have a fear of the supernatural, or a fear of God. Look at the aspen tree itself. Its leaves seem to quiver and tremble in the slightest breeze, so amazingly like the negative state of mind it treats.

The positive vibration of Aspen is *Fearlessness*. The aspen tree has both male and female flowers. The males are gray, the females smaller and green-gray. It blooms from February to early April.

Red Chestnut
Indication: Fear and Overconcern for Loved Ones
In this state we experience an overwhelming concern for those we love. We are fearful for them and we worry that something terrible will happen, and we anticipate misfortune. We feel that somehow it is our responsibility to make sure others are safe. We never seem able to rest our fears.

We all worry about our loved ones at times. When they are ill or having a hard time, of course we care and feel concern. The extreme expressions of natural concern need treatment— the mother who is constantly afraid something will happen to her child and is in a state of stress until she walks in the door, or the wife who is sure the worst has happened to her husband when he's not home on time. In these cases, Red Chestnut is indicated.

I had as a client a mother, who was dealing with the extreme Red Chestnut state. She was constantly in a state of fear over her only son's welfare. He had just starting driving and was allowed to use the car on Saturday nights. She was unable to sleep until he came home, and she fretted and worried until she heard the car in the driveway.

Once she used Red Chestnut, things changed dramatically for her. Several weeks later she called to tell me how amazed she was at the difference Red Chestnut had made in her life. Her worry and concern for her son had eased up so much that she no longer waited up for him. Her extreme fear for his safety was no longer a stressful issue for her.

The positive vibration of Red Chestnut is *Solicitude*. The red chestnut tree's flowers are deep red, blooming in late May and June.

ESSENCES FOR UNCERTAINTY

Cerato

Indication: Uncertainty in Decision-Making
Do you lack confidence in your own wisdom and intuition in making decisions for yourself? Do you constantly seek the advice of others whom you feel are more capable than you? Do you collect opinions from a number of others, weigh their advice, and then choose from among these before you can decide what to do? And do you often realize, after the fact, that your own feelings were really the best?

This is the description of the Cerato state, in which we lack confidence in decision-making. In truth, only you know what is best for yourself. When in the Cerato state, people feel uncertain about their own choices.

The positive vibration of Cerato is *Inner Certainty*. Cerato has bright blue flowers, and blooms from August to early October.

Scleranthus

Indication: Vacillation

Do you vacillate over making choices, finding it impossible to select just one? When confronted with two major choices, do you repeatedly swing back and forth from one to the other? This is truly a dilemma for any of us in this state. Which one do we pick, and is it the right choice? Maybe not, so let's change our minds…and on it goes.

I have counseled a number of women who were at a point in their lives where they needed to decide whether to continue with their careers or to take some time off to start a family. There was a strong desire for both, bringing up a great deal of uncertainty and causing them much stress. Once they used Scleranthus they were able to make the decision that was right for them, resolving their conflicting emotions.

The Scleranthus state is one of imbalance where we swing back and forth. We vacillate, instead of making choices; in this state, our emotions, too, can seem to swing back and forth—we feel up one minute and down the next. Scleranthus would be one flower essence to consider for those coping with mood swings.

The Scleranthus state is epitomized by Hamlet's famed soliloquy, "To be or not to be…"; that character is a poignant example of the indecisive Scleranthus state of mind. Cherry Plum would also be indicated for Hamlet's thoughts of suicide and Star of Bethlehem for his grief over his father's death.

The positive vibration of Scleranthus is *Balance*. Scleranthus has green flowers without petals, and blooms from late May to September.

Gentian

Indication: Discouragement Due to Setbacks and Delays

Do you lose faith when setbacks and delays frustrate you? Do you become despondent when things seem stuck? When these feelings arise, you have moved into the Gentian state. You may begin to feel, "Oh, what's the use, things never seem to work out the way I planned," and begin to think about giving up. Depression is likely to set in when this happens often, leaving us tired and discouraged. In this state we lose our faith in the process of life. We are so wrapped up in our personal plan that we forget that there is a greater plan at work—God's plan. We need to know that, first, there is a reason for everything that happens to us whether we understand what it is or not; second, everything happens for our highest good, as hard as it may be to trust this. It is only with unconditional faith that we can get through this life without feeling discouraged when things seem to go wrong.

I want to share with you a fabulous story that aptly depicts the positive Gentian state.

In a distant village in some far away land, lived two neighboring farmers, Joseph and Simon. One day, Joseph's horses broke loose and ran away. When Simon learned of this calamity, feeling bad for his friend, he went to offer his regrets. To this Joseph stoically replied," You never know."

And it then came to pass on the very next day, as luck would have it, Joseph's horses not only returned home, but following behind was a herd of wild horses. Joseph now had twice as many horses as before. Simon, upon learning of this stroke of good fortune proceeded to congratulate Joseph. However, as before, Joseph only replied, "You never know."

And so it was after the passing of several more days, Joseph's eighteen-year-old son, while training one of the new horses, was thrown and broke his leg. Simon, after learning of this tragic incident, paid his condolences for what seemed an unfortunate turn of events. Joseph, as before, seemed unperturbed and again replied, "You never know."

It soon came to pass several weeks later, while Joseph's son was recovering from his broken leg, war was declared by a neighboring village. All the young men of our farmer's village were enlisted to join forces against the enemy and do battle.

Now, as luck would have it, Joseph's son, with his broken leg, was unfit to fight. And thus remained safe at home. Simon, caught up with excitement for his friend's good fortune, rushed over to congratulate him. And true to form the only comment that Joseph made was, "You never know"...

And the truth is often that we never do know why things happen or don't happen. What we need to remember, however, is to trust that the right and perfect thing is always happening—and keep the faith.

The positive vibration of Gentian is *Faith*. Gentian's flowers are purple violet flowers and bloom from August to early October.

Gorse

Indication: Hopelessness

In the Gorse state we move into a deeper depression than found in the Gentian state. Here we experience loss of hope, and feel no more can be done for us. We feel our despondency deeply, with great sadness and despair. This can bring some people to the edge, and Cherry Plum may be indicated for control of possible impulsive actions that could be self-destructive.

Recently, I have been working with a client who has been taking antidepressant medication. She was distressed over the side effects she was experiencing with this medication. She had heard about the Bach Flower Essences and wondered if they would be able to help with her depression and her need of antidepressant medication.

I advised that she tell her doctor she was going to be working with the Bach Flower Essences, and that he monitor the medication he had given her and slowly decrease the dosage. I explained to her that it could be dangerous to stop her antidepressants abruptly. It would be safer to work with her doctor in this situation. She agreed, and over several months had her dosage reduced while taking the Bach Flower Essences. Gorse was one of the essences she had chosen. She is now nearly off antidepressants and just about free of all the side effects, and is very excited over the effectiveness of the Bach Flower Essences in relieving her depression.

The positive vibration of Gorse is *Hope*. Gorse has bright pale yellow flowers and blooms from late March to early June.

Hornbeam

Indication: Low Vitality

Do you wake up in the morning feeling tired, wishing you could roll over and go back to sleep? Has your get up and go deserted you? Once you begin your day, does your energy return? For this so-called "Monday morning feeling," Hornbeam is the indicated flower essence. The lack of vitality you're feeling in the Hornbeam state is, surprisingly, more on a mental than a physical level; there may be boredom under the surface. Hornbeam, for this reason, is also helpful for procrastination. A need for strengthening the body, as occurs in body builders who feel a lack of strength, is another nuance of the Hornbeam state that may indicate the need for this essence.

The positive vibration of Hornbeam is *Inner Vitality*. Hornbeam has both male and female flowers of yellow on the same tree and blooms in April and May.

Wild Oat

Indication: Uncertain of Life Path

Dr. Bach referred to this flower essence as "the Path Finder." When we are uncertain as to what our path in life is, Wild Oat is indicated. We may be exploring several different careers and not really sure which way to go. We may be involved in a career, yet feel unfulfilled on some level or find our heart is not in it. Dr. Bach stressed the importance of doing the work we have come here to do. When we are not in alignment with our life's purpose, we are out of harmony with our soul. As a result, we may find ourselves facing disease down the road. Wild Oat will facilitate being in tune with your mission in life when there is uncertainty.

The positive vibration of Wild Oat is *Purposefulness*. Wild Oat is a tall grass with flowering heads like the true oat and blooms in July and August.

ESSENCES FOR INSUFFICIENT INTEREST IN PRESENT CIRCUMSTANCES

Clematis

Indication: Not Being in the Present Moment

Do you find yourself lost in daydreams a bit too often? Do you often feel ungrounded, a little spacey, forget things, and feel unable to concentrate due to lack of interest? Is sleep a refuge for you, with napping during the day? These are the earmarks of the Clematis state. These individuals are often quite creative, yet are unable to make practical use of their talents. They live more in the future than in the present moment, not quite satisfied with today.

The quintessential dreamer, Don Quixote, is my favorite Clematis portrait. This flower essence is also highly effective with children coping with learning disabilities. They tend to daydream quite a bit as well as having difficulty in concentrating. Clematis helps to ground them.

The positive vibration of Clematis is *Creative Idealism.* Clematis has creamy white flowers and blooms from July through September.

Honeysuckle

Indication: Living in the Past

We were caught up in the future in the Clematis state; we are lost in the past in the Honeysuckle state. We seem to be stuck in past times, whether they are pleasant reminiscences of the good old days, or difficult memories that cause pain. We lose touch with the present and are unable to move forward in our lives. Many elderly folk fall into the Honeysuckle state as partners and friends pass on—they long for times past and are no longer living in the present. This is certainly understandable, yet definitely not healthy.

With divorce, there is also a hanging on to what used to be. Honeysuckle assists in releasing us from the past and allows us to see that life is still vital. Honeysuckle is also indicated for small children struggling with separation anxiety as well as bouts of homesickness.

Judy Garland, in her role as Dorothy in *The Wizard of Oz,* portrayed the Honeysuckle state so beautifully with the clicking of her ruby red shoes and murmuring repeatedly, "There's no place like home."

The positive vibration of Honeysuckle is the *Capacity for Change.* Honeysuckle has bright red flowers and blooms from June through August.

Wild Rose

Indication: Apathy and Resignation

Apathy and resignation are the benchmarks of the Wild Rose state. A person has accepted his lot in life. He feels as though nothing can be done to change his situation, and no attempt is made to do so. An air of resignation takes over—no effort is made to improve things. It is as though the very spark of life has just about gone out. This is not a state of depression, however. You notice a flat affect with these individuals: there are neither signs of sadness, nor any signs of joy. Nothing seems to matter anymore. A numbness sets in. There is a surrender to what is wrongly perceived as the inevitable. This state can be clearly distinguished among prisoners of war, individuals diagnosed with terminal diseases, and victims of abuse, to note several illustrations of this state. In such circumstances indifference and passivity are pervasive.

The positive vibration of Wild Rose is *Inner Motivation*. Wild Rose has flowers of either white or pink and blooms in June and July.

Olive

Indication: Extreme Exhaustion

For those who feel totally exhausted as a result of difficult emotionally and/or physically draining experiences that have totally sapped vitality, Olive is indicated. The Olive state is a deeper energy depletion than the Hornbeam state. Total exhaustion is definitive here on all levels.

Certain circumstances often bring on the Olive state: recovering from surgery or an accident, energy depletion during or after the birthing process, coping with a life-threatening illness, struggling emotionally with any major loss in life, such as the death of a loved one, loss through divorce, a career wiped away. These all profoundly deplete one's energy resources.

The positive vibration of Olive is *Regeneration*. The olive tree's flowers are creamy white and bloom in May or June.

White Chestnut

Indication: Restless Mind, Obsessive Thinking

Do unwanted thoughts constantly assail you, repeating themselves over and over? Does it seem as though a record has gotten stuck in the same groove, making it almost impossible to concentrate and focus? Obsessive thoughts, as well as an overly busy and restless mind that doesn't allow peace and rest, are indications of the White Chestnut state. At times, you may find yourself unable to fall asleep, or waking in the middle of the night. Perhaps you wake much too early and are unable to go back to sleep. Sleeplessness can become a problem in this state, and White Chestnut is often used to help in this situation.

The positive vibration of White Chestnut is *Tranquility*. The horse or white chestnut tree is related to the red chestnut tree and is similar except in color, with its flowers predominantly white with pink, red, or yellow centers, blooming in May and June.

Mustard

Indication: Depression from an Unknown Cause

Mustard is indicated for the type of depression that comes on with no apparent reason. It's as though a dark cloud has suddenly descended and then just as suddenly disappears. This essence treats depression stemming from an unknown cause. You are unaware of what it may be that is causing this gloomy feeling. When Mustard is used, the reason underlying your depressed state surfaces. In cases of PMS as well as postpartum depression, this flower essence has proven to be most effective.

The positive vibration of Mustard is *Cheerfulness*. Mustard is a common weed throughout England, with yellow flowers that bloom from May through July.

Chestnut Bud

Indication: Failure to Learn from Past Mistakes

In the negative Chestnut Bud state, we don't seem to learn from the past. We find ourselves repeating the same old habit patterns over and over—dysfunctional patterns that do not serve us and prevent our growth. Chestnut Bud is clearly indicated in cases of co-dependency, when the desire to be in relationship is stronger than our common sense. Unable to learn from our past mistakes, we repeatedly choose partners who are not good for us. Chestnut Bud would also be indicated when we indulge in unhealthy life choices, such as drug and alcohol abuse. We may stop for a while, knowing this is unhealthy. Yet we often find ourselves drawn back into the same negative behavior.

Chestnut Bud is often used with learning-disabled children who tend to not learn as quickly as other children, and fall into unproductive study habits.

The positive vibration of Chestnut Bud is the *Capacity to Learn*. The essence for Chestnut Bud also comes from the horse chestnut tree. The bud is used to make this essence; the flower is used to make White Chestnut. The buds open in season, usually early in April.

ESSENCES FOR LONELINESS

Water Violet
Indications: Aloof, Proud
When you observe the Water Violet flower in its natural surroundings, seeing how the individual plants seem to grow miles apart from each other, you are given a clue to what the negative Water Violet state is—aloof and detached from others, loners. Water Violets are proud, gentle, and independent souls. They move through life quietly, doing their work. Sometimes their sense of pride may give them the feeling that they are a little bit better than the rest of us. They have no need to interfere in others' lives, and don't want interference from others. They'd rather be left alone, for the most part. Actor James Dean, with his reputation of being a loner, illustrates this personality type.

The Water Violets' sense of independence, detachment, and pride, when taken to the extreme, often builds a wall around them that others are reluctant to broach. After a while a sense of loneliness, which is actually self-imposed, begins to be felt. No one is an island. No one can grow in isolation. It is only in relationship that growth is truly possible. Water Violets have many special gifts to share—and humanity has great need of them.

The positive vibration of Water Violet is *Humility*. Water Violet is an aquatic plant with pale mauve flowers that have yellow centers, blooming in May and June.

Impatiens
Indication: Lack of Patience

Would you rather work alone because you easily lose patience— with others slower than yourself, or with life itself, when things seem to drag? Do you find that yesterday isn't even soon enough? Are you always "pushing the river" to get things done?

Most of us can relate to the negative Impatiens state, for we experience great stress, tension, and irritability in keeping up with our lives. Time becomes our enemy when we forget to take time to enjoy just being alive. Impatiens essence is often used to treat hyperactivity and attention deficit in children.

The positive vibration of Impatiens is *Patience*. In making the Impatiens flower essence, only the pale mauve flowers are used. It blooms from July to September.

Heather
Indication: Self-involvement

This flower essence is indicated for those who, in order to share their prolific worries and concerns, need constant companionship. Heather is preoccupied only with his own issues and finds it hard to listen to others. Friends and relations often find this a drain on their energy and begin to avoid the Heather individual.

A vicious cycle develops, with the Heather's neediness and others' avoidance.

Although Heather is a definite personality type, there are times in our lives—times of crisis—when our need to unburden our troubles can temporarily take on a Heather-like quality. This essence may then be indicated.

The positive vibration of Heather is *Empathy*. Heather's flowers are pink and purple and bloom in August and September.

ESSENCES FOR OVERSENSITIVITY TO INFLUENCES AND IDEAS

Agrimony
Indication: Denial and Repression of Feelings
"Everything's fine," says the Agrimony. No one would suspect the pain and torment hidden beneath the cheerful face she presents to the world. She represses and denies her feelings to herself, too. She often turns to drugs, alcohol, and even food to self-medicate. (Note, however, that drug and alcohol dependency is not always present.) She prefers to be with others, as a distraction from her feelings. When she is alone, the TV or radio is always going. She is easily upset by arguments and confrontations, and avoids these at all costs. We can see the Agrimony profile poignantly in the life of Marilyn Monroe. She was so deeply haunted by her inner torments that only excessive use of alcohol and drugs could bring her relief.

The positive vibration of Agrimony is *Joyfulness*. Agrimony's flowers are yellow and bloom from June through August.

Centaury
Indication: Lack of Personal Boundaries, Subservient
Do you find it almost impossible to say no when asked to do someone a favor—even though it might be at your own expense? Are you easily taken advantage of, and do you have difficulty

standing up for yourself? Do you allow others to control you, and does this prevent you from caring for your own needs and following your own purpose in life? This describes the out-of-balance Centaury state.

The Centaury type is a gentle individual, sincerely wishing to serve and be of help to others. He can easily become subservient in the presence of stronger individuals. He has difficulty in setting personal boundaries and is in danger of becoming a doormat. This is detrimental to the development of his own soul. In his great desire to serve, he forgets to serve himself as well. Each of us needs to honor our personal needs, too, rather than constantly sacrifice them to the demands of others. There is a time and place to serve others, and there is a time and place to serve self. If we are always giving ourselves away, what is then left to give? If we don't take care of ourselves, eventually we won't be able to take care of others either.

In a recent Bach Flower consultation a woman came to me in an extremely out-of-balance Centaury and Agrimony state. She had a very difficult time in speaking up for herself, and shared how she allowed herself to be constantly taken advantage of. She was a very loving and gentle person with a great heart. It was her nature to be very giving and kind. But she now realized she was hurting herself by putting her own needs aside to serve and please others.

She had a hard time being in touch with her feelings, which she tended to repress by keeping constantly busy. She knew she held a great deal of pain inside, yet feared she would be overwhelmed if she allowed it to surface. She was also dealing with hypertension, and was on medication. I felt it would probably take several months for an emotional shift to take place, as her issues were long-standing and deeply ingrained in her personality.

Once she began her flower essence therapy, it took four or five months before she noticed profound changes taking place.

She told me her boss was beside himself as she began to take her personal power back, no longer going along with all his demands. She had also decided to begin psychotherapy, to process some of the deep-seated emotionally charged issues of her childhood that she felt needed to finally be released. Before my very eyes she was moving into both the positive Centaury and Agrimony states.

After about six months, her blood pressure had returned to normal and her doctor, who was very surprised, took her off her medications. The emotional healing had evidently begun to affect her physical body.

Dr. Bach did not develop his flower essences to cure primarily physical disease. They were meant to treat and overcome the negative emotional and mental links of disease and thus allow the obstructed life energy—the true source of healing—to manifest itself once again in the healing process. The essences have their greatest effect, and fulfill their most important role, as a preventative—they balance the underlying personality disharmonies so physical disease can never manifest.

When healing takes place on the emotional and mental levels, it is possible that disease which has already manifested on the physical level may also be healed. According to Dr. Bach, "As the Herbs heal our fears, our anxieties, our worries, our faults and our failings, it is these we must seek, and then the disease, no matter what it is, will leave us."

The positive vibration of Centaury is *Self-Determination*. Centaury's flowers are pale pink and bloom from June to September.

Walnut
Indication: Easily Influenced by Others
This flower essence is one of the most versatile of the thirty-eight individual flower essences. Dr. Bach called Walnut the "Link-Breaker." It is indicated for all transitions in life, including

teething, puberty, leaving home, becoming independent and entering a career, marriage, the birth of children, divorce, the empty-nest syndrome, retirement, and aging. Change is usually an uncomfortable experience. Going from the known to the unknown is not easy for most of us. Walnut facilitates the process of moving on, helping us to break the links to the old as we open to the new.

Walnut's energy also protects us from the influence of others. We may have set our course in life only to find that a parent, or some other strong individual we admire, has attempted to dissuade us. Walnut will help us be true to ourselves and to our ideas and ideals; to chart our own course without allowing others to influence us.

Dr. Bach himself was a Walnut type. Despite the medical profession's threats to take away his license because they considered his practice of medicine unorthodox, he would not allow them to dissuade him from his course.

The positive vibration of Walnut is *Unaffectedness*. The walnut tree's flowers are green. Both male and female flowers appear on the same tree. They bloom from April to late May.

Holly

Indication: Hatred, Suspicion, Envy, and Jealousy

Initially, it may be hard to recognize when we are in the negative Holly state. Its indications of hatred, envy, jealousy, suspicion, and revenge are usually pushed under the table for most of us. It is not very comfortable to own up to having any of these negative feelings. Yet most of us have experienced the Holly state at some time or another. If we are honest with ourselves, we know this.

In the Holly personality type, sadly, the heart has been closed. Every child born into this world desires to give and receive love. If this is denied, she will experience great pain and disappointment and eventually close off in defense of self. The need for love is then repressed, because love is unavailable. Love's opposite manifestations—hatred, revenge, envy, jealousy, suspicion, and a profound sense of separation from others—may arise from repressed need. This state has the potential for the development of serious disease; if left unchecked, it may have more unhealthy potential than any other state.

It may be difficult for us to have compassion and empathy for murderers and their ilk, extreme examples of the out-of-balance Holly types. While we would not condone their actions, we would see with different eyes if we understood what brought them to this state. Individuals who have been emotionally or physically abused as young children have potential need for Holly. The sense of trust has most likely been stifled, stemming from deep-seated feelings of betrayal towards those who were charged with their care and protection. It is very difficult, however, to touch these feelings of anger and outrage now buried deeply within. The need to love their parents and/or caregivers was overwhelming, and was necessary for survival. And so, what was perceived as dangerous feelings have been repressed.

These toxic emotions must eventually be brought into the light of consciousness for release. If they are not, the ability to love and be loved will continue to be hampered, and potential for the manifestation of disease will be created. Dr. Bach stated that Holly protects us from all that is not unconditional love.

The positive potential of Holly is *Unconditional Love*. The holly tree has fragrant small white flowers tinged with pink; they bloom in May and June.

ESSENCES FOR DESPONDENCY AND DESPAIR

Larch
Indication: Low Self-worth
Do you suffer from feelings of low self-esteem, lack self-worth, and believe you can never measure up to others? Do you not

even try to succeed, because you lack confidence in yourself and feel you can never succeed where others do? In the Larch state we are out of touch with our individual uniqueness and specialness. We have lost sight of our own distinctive gifts and talents.

Each of us has come into this world with a special purpose that only we can fulfill. And we have been equipped with the resources to accomplish this if we would only realize it. We have forgotten our divine heritage as a child of God. Truly, in God's eyes not one of us is seen as having a greater or lesser value. Let us recognize and value ourselves, and what we have come to share, as our Creator does.

The Larch state usually has its roots in our childhood. Good parenting is not a subject taught in school, and infants do not come with instructions. Many of us have been raised without the nurturance of self-worth. We were told we were "bad little boys" (or girls) as we were scolded for merely attempting to learn about life. This began, typically, at a very early age, when we were vulnerable, took everything to heart, and accepted much as implicit truth. As a result, most of us grow up with more or less deficient self-esteem. It is vital to our health that we learn to value ourselves and finally re-program those old tapes.

Larch is often indicated for children with learning disabilities, for whom low self-esteem can be a major issue. Many of these children are aware that they are different and, unfortunately, internalize this as a lack. This often produces feelings of inferiority, and they begin to give up. Gentian would also be indicated when feelings of despair are present, caused by any setback to their learning.

The positive vibration of Larch is *Self-Confidence*. The larch tree produces both male and female flowers. Male flowers are yellow; female flowers are red. They bloom in late March and April.

Pine

Indication: Self-blame and Guilt

Pine individuals are perfectionists, very critical of themselves, never satisfied with their accomplishments, and feeling they could have done a better job. A sense of guilt underlies this perceived lack of personal perfection. This personality characteristic was often instilled by parents who were overly demanding in what they expect from their child. They send the message (consciously or unconsciously) that what their child has accomplished is never "good enough." No matter what he does, a sense of underlying disapproval remains. Thus, as he grows into adulthood this feeling is internalized and eventually manifests as a drive for perfection. His inner child continues to search for the approval it never received.

Curiously, the feelings of guilt that have been internalized, of not being good enough, spill over onto the mistakes of others. The Pine somehow feels responsible or at fault for the mistake, often apologizing for others' errors that have nothing to do with him.

Several years ago, a dear friend of mine was showing strong indications of the Pine type. She not only was very self-critical, but was always apologizing when anything went wrong, though it had nothing to do with any of her actions. One day I knocked over my coffee cup, spilling its contents. She jumped up exclaiming, "Oh, I'm so sorry," as if somehow it had been her fault. I was surprised at her response and told her so. I asked if she realized that she had this tendency to take the blame for others. She agreed that this was a pattern she recognized in herself. With my knowledge of the Bach Flowers, how could I not help a friend? To this day she uses Pine, and her self-deprecating behavior has disappeared.

The positive vibration of Pine is *Forgiveness*. The pine tree has both male (clusters of small yellow balls) and female (red cone-shaped) flowers that bloom in May.

Elm

Indication: Overwhelmed

Are you overwhelmed by all your responsibilities, feeling unable to fulfill them? Have you put too much on your plate? Elm is usually a temporary state, one that surfaces when we take on too much. Usually those who suffer from the Elm state are responsible individuals who have unwittingly overburdened themselves. This is not an issue of lack of responsibility, but one of too much responsibility. Elm helps us set priorities among our duties, and brings awareness of our limits. One individual can only accomplish so much at any given time.

The positive vibration of Elm is *Right Responsibility*. The elm tree's flowers appear before the leaves and are small reddish brown clusters, blooming in February or March.

Sweet Chestnut

Indication: Extreme Anguish

The negative Sweet Chestnut state is profound despair. We have reached the limits of our endurance, and have gone well beyond the Gorse state of hopelessness. In Sweet Chestnut we have entered into the dark night of the soul. The light of life itself is nowhere to be found. The anguish that is experienced in this state is beyond words, as though our very soul is facing annihilation. The suffering one feels is so deep that it seems that nothing could possibly ease the pain—not even death itself.

I recently treated a client with Sweet Chestnut for her anguish over the attempted suicide of her son. It was uncertain whether he would survive through the night. She had been a past client and called me from the hospital for help, on the verge of falling apart. She had remembered how helpful the essences had been before and somehow had the presence of mind during this crisis to contact me. I made arrangements for her to receive Sweet Chestnut immediately. The next day she shared with me how this flower essence brought her relief, and helped hold her together while waiting through the night for a change in her son's condition. We were thankful that he had come through his ordeal and would recover.

The positive vibration of Sweet Chestnut is *Release*. The sweet chestnut tree has both male (catkins) and female (green) flowers which bloom in July.

Star of Bethlehem
Indication: Grief, Shock, Trauma

Called the "Comforter" by Dr. Bach, Star of Bethlehem brings relief from grief, shock, and trauma. This flower essence is indicated for treating the after-effects of all shock and trauma, physical or emotional. Star would be indicated after an accident or operation; for victims of rape, incest, and other forms of abuse; upon learning of the death of a loved one; and for any loss we may suffer that brings grief and bereavement.

Whenever we are traumatized, the cells of the body record and hold these traumas. We retain within our cellular structure the memory of all instances of trauma beginning with, and including, the moment of birth. In cases of Post-Traumatic Stress Disorder (PTSD), we can see the persistent re-experiencing of a traumatic event that took place in the past. Although the original trauma has long passed, the individual suffering from PTSD has recurrent and intrusive recollections of the event, or distressing dreams in which the event is replayed. Star has the ability to move into the cellular memory itself, and release these painful memories to facilitate the healing process on the deepest level.

As with the case of PTSD, any other traumatic experiences that are held within may also become symptomatic in the development of disease at a later time. As nearly everyone experiences trauma to some degree in the course of life, Star is one flower essence we all may need sometime.

The positive vibration of Star of Bethlehem is *Restoration*. Star of Bethlehem has bright white flowers that bloom from April to June.

Willow

Indication: Bitterness, Resentment

Do you find yourself blaming others for your problems? Do you see yourself as a victim in many instances, and do not see the part you may have played in manifesting the outcome? The out-of-balance Willow individual is filled with resentment and bitterness towards others she feels have wronged her, or against life's injustices. Things do come to us that seem unfair, and that we feel we don't deserve. With our limited understanding, with our finite minds, it is not always possible to understand why bad things happen to good people. This is not to condone the hurtful action of others. Yet, there is a purpose regardless of our ability to comprehend it.

The grand scheme of life itself gives us opportunities to grow beyond our trials. When we perceive that all that comes to us has merely been a lesson, and then make the effort to learn from this, we are strengthened beyond measure. If we choose, instead, to hold on to bitterness and resentment, we are hurting ourselves much more deeply than we realize. If we continue to hold on to these highly toxic emotions, they will greatly affect our health in the long run.

It is said that we attract to ourselves the people and lessons we need, and all are merely teachers for us. It is crucial that we release blame towards others, take responsibility for our lives, and see all that transpires as a catalyst for our personal growth.

The positive vibration of Willow is *Personal Responsibility*. The willow tree bears either male or female flowers (long green catkins), exclusively. These blossom during April or May.

Oak

Indication: Endurance Despite Hardship

Oak personalities are long-suffering individuals, enduring through whatever trials are presented to them, rarely giving up or asking others for help. The oak is one of the strongest trees, and the Oak type is one of the strongest people. The major issue of the Oak is his tendency to drive himself into the ground. He can become exhausted because he never knows when to quit, and pushes himself too hard. Even Oaks need to take a breather from time to time, and not take life so seriously. Unfortunately, many do not have "vacation" in their vocabulary, and consider "play" a four-letter word. The needs of the physical body for rest and relaxation are too often ignored. This will take its toll at some point. Learning that life is not all work, and that play is important, is the lesson to be mastered by the out-of-balance Oak. Oak is also recommended for adding inner strength when enduring difficult trials.

The positive vibration of Oak is *Endurance*. The English oak, with its female flowers of small red buds and its male flowers of catkins, blooms in late April through May.

Crab Apple

Indication: Self-disgust

Individuals who are in the out-of-balance Crab Apple state are fastidious with personal hygiene and with their surroundings. They have an almost obsessive need for order and purity. They are so sensitive that even the smallest disorder disturbs their equilibrium. They may compulsively clean their homes and their bodies for an all-pervasive feeling of uncleanliness surrounds them. In the extreme, they may develop feelings of self-disgust and self-loathing, and view their bodies with disdain for whatever characteristics they may perceive as unacceptable flaws. There may also be an aversion to germs, with the fear of contamination becoming almost obsessive.

Crab Apple is the essence that brings these issues into balance, and it is known the "Cleanser." It is a most exceptional flower essence in that it comes closest to influencing the physical body itself. As we have learned, flower essences operate within the emotional and mental levels of our energetic system. Crab Apple, however, seems also to facilitate the release of toxins on the physical level. You will find Crab Apple to be helpful when coping with a cold or the flu. It is also the flower essence to consider when undergoing radiation and/or chemotherapy treatments.

We can see the negative Crab Apple personality expressed in Michael Jackson. He seems to have been dealing with feelings of self-disgust for years, from the indications given by the innumerable changes he has made to his physical appearance.

Individuals who suffer from anorexia are also in the negative Crab Apple state, obsessing over their weight. This essence is also highly recommended for victims of rape and incest. They are likely to be coping with feelings of being soiled and unclean to the very core of their beings, and they often hold deep-seated feelings of shame.

The positive vibration of Crab Apple is *Purity*. The crab apple tree has white flowers that bloom in May.

ESSENCES FOR OVER-CARE FOR WELFARE OF OTHERS

Chicory

Indication: Possessive, Manipulative

The mother (or father) hen syndrome is part of the Chicory profile. These individuals are constantly fussing over their loved ones, making sure they're doing the right thing—to the Chicory's way of thinking. They tend to be quite possessive. They always need attention and start to pout when they are ignored. Chicory types are very giving. However, there are always strings attached.

When the Chicory doesn't feel appreciated, it is common to hear her say, "After all I've done for you…." She can be quite the martyr, and manipulation is a sword she wields well, instilling guilt in others who won't cooperate with her agenda in the hope of her gaining control once again.

Chicory has the potential of a very great love, a love that gives without needing anything in return. It is the love that a mother holds for her newborn, a love she ceaselessly gives with no expectations from her helpless and totally dependent babe. And it is her joy to do so. It is only when Chicory is out of balance that her love becomes possessive and selfish. This essence has also been used most effectively with young children, as well as pets, who demand a great deal of attention.

The positive vibration of Chicory is *Selfless Love*. Chicory's blossoms are a rich blue, flowering from July to September.

Vervain

Indication: Overenthusiastic, Opinionated

Are you a high-energy individual, filled with enthusiasm and excitement? However, is it perhaps a bit too much, especially when it comes to sharing your beliefs and opinions? Do you get into arguments, never giving in, knowing you are *always* right, and refuse to listen to the other side? Do you tend to proselytize and love to stand on your soap box? But do you *only* share, in your opinion, that which is the only truth? Vervain is the essence for those who relate to the above.

Actually, Vervains, when in balance, are our greatest teachers who touch our hearts and inspire us, as did Dr. Martin Luther King. Unfortunately, when out of balance the Vervain can get a bit carried away and become a bit too rigid and inflexible in his beliefs.

I will now self-disclose and admit that I am a Vervain personality type (if you haven't already guessed). Hopefully, I am in balance most of the time. Yet, I recognize that my zeal for teaching others is always under the surface, just waiting for the right opportunity to surface. Just the other day, while I was getting some coffee in a 7-11, I noticed a woman who seemed stressed. Somehow I found myself involved in a conversation with her, and before I knew it the Bach Flowers came up. The fact that she took time to listen to me and seemed interested gave me the go-ahead. She spent the next fifteen minutes hearing a mini-lecture on Bach Flowers. I'll never know if she was just being polite or was really interested, although she did make a note of their name and asked where the essences could be purchased.

What I have just shared is a Vervain in action. We have this burning desire to help others—to teach others. We just need to make sure that others want to know about what we have to share and avoid being intrusive. Vervain also has a strong sense of justice and of what is right and fair, with a willingness to fight for the underdog. This essence is also quite helpful in cases of hyperactivity.

The positive vibration of Vervain is *Restraint*. Vervain's flowers are small blossoms of pale mauve or pink that bloom from June to September.

Vine

Indication: Domineering, Inflexible

There is inflexibility and rigidity with a Vine out of balance (as was with a Vervain). In this state, however, it is not so much a need to teach or force your personal opinion on others, or to get them to embrace and follow your beliefs. With Vine it's merely a matter of his knowing that *his* way is the *only* way, with the qualities of domination and control added on. There are no arguments with a Vine.

Throughout history we have seen examples of the negative Vine type personified in many dictators. In truth, Vines are natural leaders and the ones you want to have around during any emergency or other situation in which good leadership is needed. When in balance, they are beneficent leaders who also listen to, and take advice from, others. They realize the futility in taking total control over everything. Vine understands that no one person has the resources to do so, and is able to delegate responsibility to others. Control is no longer an issue, as it is with the out-of-balance Vine in his misuse of power and authority. Nor is the burden of taking all the responsibility upon his shoulders his alone. The gifts of Vine, including his ability to achieve success in almost anything he puts his mind to, must be put to use for the greater good of all. This essence is also quite helpful for the bossy child as well as the bossy animal.

The positive vibration of Vine is *Right Use of Authority*. Vine's flowers are green in color and bloom in early summer.

Beech

Indication: Critical, Judgmental, Intolerant

Are you easily disturbed by other people's idiosyncrasies and find yourself to be critical of others in general? Do you constantly nit-pick and always find fault? This state of being overly critical is not for oneself but directed outward towards others. In this out-of-balance Beech state, there is a prevailing sense of intolerance which may also encompass feelings of prejudice.

The Beech individual has forgotten the law of Unity—the oneness of all things. Any cruelty or wrong done to another affects our Creator as well as ourselves, bringing discord and eventually disease. No one is perfect, not even the Beech, although in her arrogance she might want to believe this.

Jesus pointed this out to the citizens who were determined to stone a women thought to be an adulteress. If there was anyone among them who had not also sinned, said Jesus, let that person cast the first stone. No one could throw a stone. Each knew himself to be guilty of some past sin. In their arrogance, these self-righteous citizens had conveniently forgotten their own imperfection. Beech is also for all degrees of intolerance and of great assistance even with PMS. During this time a woman may be more sensitive to others, as well as less tolerant.

The positive vibration of Beech is *Tolerance*. The beech tree has both male and female flowers on the same tree, blooming in April and May.

Rock Water
Indication: Self-denying

We have come to our final individual flower essence, Rock Water. This essence is indicated for those who are overly strict with themselves in following the high ideals they have set forth to live by. These individuals desire to be examples to others, although they do not push their ideals as does the Vervain type, or take a position of authority as does the Vine. In their own quiet way—by demonstration—the Rock Water type hopes to inspire others. She strives for personal perfection, but does so in such a self-denying manner that there is no joy left in her life.

It is evident that there is also a rigidity inherent in the Rock Water state, as with Vine and Vervain. However, this inflexibility is directed against the self, many times suppressing important human needs. These individuals all adhere to a strict living style, be it a personal, religious, or social discipline. We easily recognize this state in the personalities of Mother Teresa and Mahatma Gandhi—two of the most notable Rock Waters of the twentieth century.

The positive vibration of Rock Water is *Adaptability*. This is the only one of all thirty-eight flower essences that is not made from a flower. Rock Water comes from healing waters found by Dr. Bach near his home in Wales.

When you choose an essence that relates to your personality type, the essences *never* change your basic personality. This is important to remember and understand. A Rock Water remains a Rock Water, an Oak remains an Oak, and a Water Violet remains a Water Violet, as well as for all the other flower essence types. The flower essences simply re-establish balance and harmony within your personality as they dissipate the negative manifestations that are harmful to your well-being.

I cite these three examples with purpose as they are described so positively. Rock Waters, Oaks, and Water Violets may feel they do not want to lose the inherent qualities they possess. Remember that it is a question of balance. When these types or any of the others move into the negative state, the resulting discord will advance disease. Thus, in any out-of-balance state there is a need for the appropriate flower essence. Choosing your flower essence type(s) will be more thoroughly described in the next chapter.

THE COMPOSITE ESSENCE—RESCUE REMEDY

This remarkable composite of five of the thirty-eight flower essences is the only ready-made combination that Dr. Bach developed. It is used during any emergency or crisis situation that may arise and brings almost instant relief. The reaction time of the individual flower essences usually takes longer. This depends upon how long a particular issue or situation has been going on for you, and how deeply ingrained into the personality any negative emotion or state of mind may be. With long-standing issues it may take several weeks, or even months, for a response to be noticed. With any issue or negative state that is current or short-term, your response will be much quicker, perhaps within several days. Keep in mind that the Bach Flower Essences are a very individualized modality. Reaction time depends on the individual, and no specific time can be given in determining your response.

The effects of Rescue Remedy are felt within several minutes; that makes this combination unique. Fast effect is possible because the state one experiences in crises and emergencies is out of the norm. We have been thrown out of balance by a dire situation that comes upon us unexpectedly. As this imbalance is very current, the re-establishment of our system's equilibrium is immediate when Rescue is taken.

The Rescue Remedy Flower Essence Combination

• Cherry Plum for fear of loss of control
• Clematis for possible loss of consciousness or dizziness
• Impatiens for pain and tension
• Rock Rose for panic and terror
• Star of Bethlehem for grief, shock, and trauma

There is also Rescue Remedy cream, which contains one additional essence, Crab Apple. As Rescue cream is used topically for many different situations, including scratches, cuts, insect bites, and even for burns and bruises, Crab Apple was added for its cleansing vibration.

The many uses for both Rescue liquid and cream are as phenomenal as is their efficacy. These are two preparations that no one should ever be without. If you use no other essences, at least please consider these. You will be amazed at the many unexpected times you will have need of them; you will be grateful to have them immediately available. From my personal experience alone, not even considering how extraordinarily helpful they have been for my clients, I believe that no medicine cabinet, purse, or glove compartment should be without them. You never know when any unexpected emergency or crisis situation will arise.

Rescue is indicated for use after receiving any news that is shocking and trauma-producing, such as hearing of the death of a loved one, being dismissed from a job, or going through a divorce. Rescue also relieves the following: anxiety and panic over a dental or doctor appointment, public speaking, feeling dizzy and faint, experiencing nausea, witnessing an accident or being involved in one (or a near miss, especially while driving), being upset by a quarrel or argument, fear of flying, going for a job interview or being called in by the boss, general feelings of stress that develop in the normal course of the day on the job or at home, panic attacks, and for many other upsetting or crisis situations too numerous to mention.

Rescue cream, aside from the uses previously cited, can also be used to soothe sore nipples after breast-feeding and is excellent in preventing stretch marks during pregnancy, both on the abdomen and the breasts. Simply apply the cream to these areas in the later stages of pregnancy. Rescue is also a wonderful help in soothing tired or irritated eyes, and both the liquid and/or cream can be applied. Place four drops of the liquid concentrate in one-half glass of water. Drop two cotton balls in the solution and then apply as a compress to the eyes for fifteen minutes. Then apply the cream, or use the cream alone if you don't have the time to relax with the compress. Blemishes as well as rashes are also quickly reduced with the use of this outstanding cream.

As you have just seen, the uses for Rescue are innumerable. It is also a most remarkable essence for treatment of animals, especially when you are not sure of the particular emotions that may be out of balance with your pet. Rescue will assist in the alleviation of whatever stress your pet may be undergoing. Don't be surprised that the flower essences are also used with animals—any living system, including plants, can benefit from the use of flower essences when indicated. Information on treating animals and plants are included in the next chapter.

The essences work even more quickly with our pets, who carry a lot less emotional baggage than we do. Flower essences are not placebos; mind over matter is not possible with our pets, yet flower essences produce positive changes in them. Bach Flowers help us regardless of whether we believe in them.

It is never possible to overdose with your use of Bach Flowers. Rescue, or any of the other flower essences, may be taken as often as needed. One day, you may have a Rescue Remedy day and need to use Rescue every few hours. Should this happen, don't be concerned. Use it as often as you need. You will never experience any side effects with the use of flower essences. Uppermost in Dr. Bach's mind was that his essences would be absolutely gentle and totally safe for use by anyone. And he personally tested each and every one on himself to ensure their gentleness and safety.

As we end this chapter, I leave you with two extraordinary experiences I have had with Rescue when I presented Bach Flower weekend seminars countrywide. I had to often travel by plane, and on one particular flight, I was seated next to a young woman and her cat. The animal had to be placed in a wire cage under the seat, according to the airline rules and regulations. As you can imagine, the cat was terrified in its strange surroundings and meowed pitifully.

Once we lifted off, I took Rescue cream from my purse, introduced myself, and proceeded to tell the young woman about how helpful Rescue would be in calming her cat. She took the tube from my hand and read the label, not quite sure what to do. After all, I was a stranger. Evidently the cat's distress finally prompted her to agree. She allowed me to place some Rescue cream on the cat's nose. Of course, she licked it off as I'd hoped. I used the cream rather than the liquid, as the concentrate has a high alcohol content. I knew the cat would refuse it. The cream has the same ingredients as the liquid, is safe to ingest, and would be just as effective in relaxing the cat.

Within ten minutes the cat stopped crying, curled herself into a ball and went to sleep for the duration of the flight. The young woman was amazed—and delighted. She wrote down the name of Rescue and inquired where it was sold. It seems God watches over cats too! Was it only an accident that I happened to be seated next to this frightened kitty?

On another flight several weeks later, a terrified woman who had never flown before had the good fortune (in my opinion) to sit next to me! Her face was white as she clutched onto the armrests of her seat, and her breathing was shallow. She was not a happy camper as we headed for the clouds.

Maybe if I were a Water Violet, I would have kept quiet. But the Vervain in me made me do it! I told her I noticed she seemed extremely nervous. She said this was her first time flying and that, yes, she was extremely nervous. I took out my bottle of Rescue and introduced her to the Bach Flowers. I asked if she'd like to try some in her apple juice. She first looked at the label and then looked at me, deciding whether or not to trust a total stranger.

Well, it seemed her panic over flying was stronger than any mistrust towards me, and she quickly agreed. It was amazing to watch the changes that took place in the next five minutes. Right before my eyes, her color returned and her breathing slowed. Little by little, her grip loosened on the armrests as the Rescue was taking effect. She turned to me in total surprise and said she couldn't believe how calm she felt. As this was not her only flight, having to change planes to continue on to her final destination, I asked if she'd like to keep my bottle of Rescue for the rest of her trip. Without hesitation she gratefully accepted my offer!

On a more serious note, as you can see from my personal experience, you never know when the need for Rescue will arise. An unexpected crisis can occur at any time, either to you or those around you, where you might need to use Rescue Remedy or share it with others.

The next chapter helps you use the flower essences—with maximum effectiveness.

4.

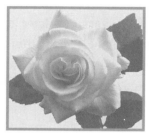

Traditional Bach Flower Therapy

This system of treatment is the most perfect that has been given to mankind within living memory. It has the power to cure disease…No science, no knowledge is necessary, apart from the simple methods described herein; and they who will obtain the greatest benefit from this God-sent Gift will be those who keep it pure as it is…for everything in Nature is simple.

—*Edward Bach,* The Twelve Healers

Thus far we have explored 1) the concept of vibrational healing, 2) Dr. Bach's personal insights into what constitutes health and the participation of every individual—or "soul" in the process of health, and 3) the indications for each of the thirty-nine flower essences that relate to the negative emotions, states of mind, and personality types that each flower essence addresses. We are now ready to proceed with the "how to" aspect of the use and practice of the Bach Flowers.

BACH FLOWER USAGE

Once you have established which of the flower essences you

need, it is critical that you are prepared to make a firm commitment to use them consistently to experience their maximum benefit. It is also important to know that a wrong selection can do *no* harm, although it will not help either. If after at least four to six weeks you find that no change is taking place, you may not be using the appropriate essences for your situation, or you are not taking them consistently enough.

The suggested dosage is *two* drops of each of the single flower essences or *four* drops of the composite formula, Rescue. They may be taken directly from the concentrate bottle and dropped under the tongue, or placed into half a glass of water, juice, tea, coffee, or other liquid. Each sip is considered a dose. They are to be taken a minimum of *four* times daily. However, as there is no danger of overdosing, you may use your essences as often as you feel the need. However, taking your essences more often would be helpful, especially when just starting to use them—or changing to a new one. In this way you are flooding your system with the essences' positive vibrations for maximum efficacy. If you are taking other medication, the flower essences will not interfere with it, nor will the other medication interfere with the flower essences. Remember, they do not work in the physical body as do other medications, nor are there any side effects to be concerned over. The flower essences are so safe and gentle that many women use them during pregnancy, while nursing, and with their infants and young children. It is not recommended to administer the essences to children directly from the concentrate bottle due to the high alcohol content. You may place the drops into their juice, milk, or other liquid, or simply prepare a personal formula dilution bottle. In fact, it is generally recommended to do this for yourself also. This makes taking several essences so much easier and is also more economical. Please be assured that when making a dilution bottle, potency is not lost. The strength of the dilution preparation is equal to the concentrate.

DILUTION BOTTLE PREPARATION AND DOSAGE

To make your personal dilution bottle, you will need a one-ounce amber dropper bottle. These are available at most drug stores or wherever the flower essences are sold. Fill the bottle three-quarters full with spring water. Add two drops of each of the essences you have selected; if you are using Rescue, add four drops. To prevent spoilage, add one teaspoon of *one* of the following as a preservative: *apple cider vinegar, vegetable glycerine,* or *brandy.* Your personal formula is now ready to be used: take *four drops* under the tongue, *four times daily* at the minimum.

When it is time to refill your bottle, simply repeat the above procedure. If you are changing any of your essences, it is necessary to sterilize your bottle before proceeding, in order to remove previous essence vibrations. Simply place your bottle and dropper top in a pot of boiling water for fifteen minutes. Remove and allow to cool. The bottle is now ready to be reused. Please take care to avoid contaminating the dropper with your tongue when administering. If this happens, just rinse the dropper with hot water before replacing it back in the bottle. There is no need to refrigerate your dilution bottle or the concentrates. However, it is important to keep them in a cool, dark place to prevent spoilage.

RECOMMENDED MAXIMUM NUMBER OF FLOWER ESSENCES

It is recommended that no more than *seven* flower essences be used at any one time. Although Rescue is a composite formula, it is counted as one essence when included in your personal formula. It may seem overwhelming at first to limit your selections to only seven. Many new users find this a challenge, feeling they could use almost all thirty-eight. Select the flower essences which address your most pressing issues—those which affect you most deeply, and which are your greatest struggle.

If you find that you are unable to limit your selection to only seven you may want to make use of an *intensity scale*. This procedure consists of noting all the essences under consideration on a piece of paper and deciding which of these relates to the issues you experience on a daily basis, every few days, weekly, and so on. You will then assign a number from one to ten to each selection under consideration. The number ten represents your most intense issues and the number one indicates your least intense issues. You may need to repeat this procedure several times before you arrive at the recommended maximum of seven. Remember to choose your essences for the issues that you find the most problematic. Make a note of the ones also considered but not chosen. These essences may be selected at a later period if they are still needed.

It may also be helpful to go over your selections with someone who knows you well, perhaps a trusted friend or loving family member. They may have some insight, especially into your personality flaws that you are not aware of, and assist in bringing this to light for you. It is not uncommon for most of us to be out of touch with our negative personality traits. It is commendable, and certainly an act of courage, to be willing to be honest with ourselves and face them head on. Without awareness, it is not possible to make changes, nor is it possible to grow. Honesty and humility are necessary companions on our journey to wholeness.

FLOWER ESSENCE PRACTICE

The Bach Flowers were developed to bring balance and harmony to acute emergency situations, transient negative emotional moods, and deep-seated negative emotions, and for treating negative personality traits. In all these situations and conditions, our body's homeostasis is interrupted and we are thrown out of balance. When we remain in this state of disequilibrium, our health is threatened, either now or at some time in the future.

In this light, Bach Flowers can be seen as a preventative approach because they restore our equilibrium before any manifestation of disease can ensue. It would also seem that by treating the cause—the negative emotions and/or negative states of mind underlying the conception of disease—the disease would eventually dissipate.

It is easy for most of us to be in touch with emergency situations that arise and passing negative moods that develop in the course of everyday life. I doubt there is anyone among us who has not been thrown out of balance when these conditions manifest. It is also a simple matter to recognize the flower essences needed when this occurs. However, deep-seated negative emotions and personality traits may be more difficult to recognize within ourselves and therefore more challenging to heal. Yet, it is so important to our state of health that we attempt to make the effort to explore our deep-seated negative emotions and our character flaws in the interest of maintaining our health and to assure our emotional healing and personal growth.

Recognize the positive step you are taking as you honestly explore personality traits that do not serve your highest good— traits that prevent you from truly living in peace and harmony with yourself and others. The flower essences that relate to your personality are possibly the most important. I urge you to discover those that correlate to your personality type. There may be more than one, as we are truly complex entities.

Also search within yourself to discover what emotional wounds you may be carrying since childhood, as well as those ensuing over the years. Many of us are in need of releasing and healing these long-standing issues of the past. Holding on to them does not serve us, but continues to produce imbalance on an energetic level, and can eventually result in the creation of disease.

For the sake of your future health, I urge you to please move through them and finally let them go. The past is over and gone. It is time to bring resolution to whatever you may be holding onto in order to move forward with your life. Power is always in the present moment. It is here that we choose the light or remain in darkness. It is here that we choose life or death.

The Peeling Effect

In your use of Bach Flowers, you will discover that as you heal certain issues, other deeper, underlying issues will begin to surface and need to be healed as well. This phenomenon is referred to as the *peeling effect*. In the process of healing, it seems that we begin our healing at the outermost level. As surface issues are released—peeled away—more profound issues are then exposed beneath the top layers that then need to be addressed. We can utilize the analogy of the onion with its many layers to help in our understanding of this process.

Over the years of this life, and possibly other incarnations, we have built up layers of negative emotions and states of mind that cover the core self—the soul—which is all beauty and perfection. In doing this we have blocked our true self from expression. We have lost our connection to our divinity, rendering our personality and soul out of alignment. This is the true cause of disease. It behooves us all, in the interest of health and wholeness to free our core self, to unblock it once again so that alignment may be reinstated between the personality and the soul. We do this by peeling away the negativity that surrounds our true self, by healing our negative emotional issues and personality characteristics that prevent us from being all that we can be—all that we were intended to be by our Creator.

PERSONALITY TYPE ESSENCES

Although the personality type essence has previously been mentioned as assisting in restoring balance to our character flaws, I feel it is important to emphasize the significance of discovering your own *type* essence(s). Dr. Bach maintained that we would greatly benefit from determining those essences that related to our personality. He advised that we always use them, as these flower essences contain our unique vibrations. Even when balance has been established, it would be advantageous to continue to use our type essences for preventative purposes.

It is not surprising, in your process of becoming more in touch with yourself, to feel initially that certain essences are your type, only to discover later on that they were not. This phenomenon is directly related to the peeling effect. As we become more aware of ourselves, as our healing process deepens, our shadows are brought up to the light for recognition and release. Do your best, from where you are now, to determine your type essence(s).

Again, honesty is paramount. Delve within yourself and be willing to recognize certain attributes and characteristics you may not be proud of owning. Are you overly possessive and manipulative (Chicory)? Are you judgmental and critical of others (Beech)? Are you overly domineering and controlling (Vine)? Do you tend to escape from life and live in a fantasy world (Clematis), or are you living in the past, constantly wishing for the good old days (Honeysuckle)? Do you avoid your feelings, resorting to drugs or alcohol to mask them (Agrimony)?

With self-reflection, it is not difficult to recognize your most obvious personality traits. Again, it might be helpful to ask a close friend for help with this process of self-exploration. Don't be concerned whether your type essence will seem to change as your healing process deepens. It is only through new awareness that we may discover the next level. Only then are we ready to move forward in our continuing process of healing.

Be aware that most of the flower essences treat both *type*—a long-standing, challenging character trait inherent to our personality and *mood*, a particular emotion or state of mind that we may be experiencing during a specific time. To clarify this, let's look at several examples. Mary is a deeply shy and timid woman—a Mimulus type. Her timidity and fear have severely hampered her life. The flower essence Mimulus would be indicated as one of Mary's type essences. Or, perhaps John is coping with the fear of losing his job. His company is being downsized. He is not a shy, timid, or a normally fearful man. Yet, because of present life circumstances, he is in a state of fear. Mimulus would also be indicated for John's current emotional state.

Another example is Sally, an overly fastidious woman. She is constantly worried that her home will become unsanitary, spending an inordinate amount of time and energy in cleaning. The flower essence, Crab Apple, would be indicated as one of Sally's type essences. Or perhaps Jane is having difficulty dealing with her body image. She is seven months pregnant and has gained thirty pounds. Every time she looks in the mirror, she is filled with self-loathing at the change in her figure. Body image had never been a problem before this. Crab Apple would also be indicated for Jane's present state of mind.

As a final illustration, although Holly is a definite type essence for individuals who have deep-seated hatred, are suspicious, jealous, or envious, there may come a time in anyone's life when a Holly state is triggered. This can occur during a divorce, heated argument, or any situation that brings up feelings of hatred at being mistreated.

As you can see from these examples, you never really know what issues may come up for you as you journey through life. Having all thirty-eight flower essences, especially Rescue Remedy, at your fingertips would certainly be worth your consideration.

ALCOHOL SENSITIVITY

Although the flower essences contain a significant amount of alcohol (in the concentrate form), individuals who are alcohol sensitive may also use them. Of course, it is recommended that they not take them by mouth directly from the concentrate. It is best to dilute the essences in a half glass of water or other liquid, or to prepare a dilution bottle as previously instructed. And, of course, *never* choose brandy as the preservative.

Another suggestion is to use the essences topically by applying them to the pulse points of the body. It would be a good idea to first make a dilution bottle before applying directly upon the skin. You may also add the essences to a spray bottle and mist the room, thereby getting their effect in this way as well. Please be advised, anyone taking the medication Antabuse should never use the Bach Flowers, nor any other substance that contains alcohol, as this medication produces an adverse affect when combined with alcohol.

REACTION TIME

It is not possible to determine how long you may need to take a particular flower essence. We are all unique, and therefore one individual's response will be different than another's. Only you can ascertain when a particular essence has resolved your situation. When you no longer feel the need to continue with any essence you are taking, simply stop. If you notice the negative feelings resurfacing, then resume taking that specific essence, as the release has not been completed. You may need to continue a while longer.

You may discover that some flower essences will only be needed on a short-term basis. You may use particular essences only once and never need them again. You may use others long-term—for months, even years. This depends on how deeply ingrained they have become within the personality, thus increasing the length of time for your healing process. And type essences are truly for the long haul—for the rest of your life, actually. If you take Dr. Bach's recommendation, you will continue using your type essences throughout your life.

As previously mentioned, you will most likely discover the peeling effect taking place at some point in your Bach Flower therapy. As your surface issues are healed and peeled away, you will find your deeper level issues now rising up to be healed as well. It would seem that, in these uncertain and stressful times, I doubt that there would ever be a period when the need for Bach Flowers would be absent.

Retrospective Quality

Because Dr. Bach intentionally developed his flower essences to be extremely gentle and safe, you will often be unaware of the subtle positive changes that take place immediately. Many users report that they realize the positive effects several days after the fact. They become aware of the emotional or mental shift that the flower essences have produced for them, only in retrospect. Or perhaps someone close to them brings this to their attention by commenting on the difference noticed in their behavior or character.

Possible Emotional Reactions to Flower Essences

There are no side effects produced by Dr. Bach's flower essences. However, it is important to mention that, on rare occasions, there are some individuals who may experience their negative emotional state intensifying somewhat when they first take the flower essences. This is actually caused by the release of the negative state itself. This intensification lasts for a very short time, from several hours to a day or two, at the most. Let me emphasize again that this is very rare. If you are among the very few in this category, you need to know what is taking place so as not to be concerned. If you find these intensified emotions too uncomfortable and are unable to let the healing process of release take its course at this time, discontinue the flower essence that is causing you discomfort. If needed, Rescue Remedy, taken as often as necessary, can be used to ease this situation. However, if you decide to push through this experience, you may also use Rescue, along with your other flower essences, to help relieve this short-term emotional intensification.

In the past, I witnessed this situation firsthand, at a Bach Flower weekend seminar I was presenting. As I was speaking on a Sunday morning, one of the participants dissolved into tears. At the close of Saturday's session, the group had been asked to choose one flower essence to work with overnight. This gives each student personal experience in flower essence use. The next morning, students share their responses with the group. Many report having unusual dreams or receiving some new personal insight.

This particular Sunday morning, as the group began sharing their experiences, one of the students started sobbing. Immediately I knew that she was experiencing an intensification. Some old emotional issue was now being released by the flower essence she had selected at the close of yesterday's session. I also had a gut feeling as to which essence she had taken—Star of Bethlehem.

I gently inquired as to which Bach Flower she had chosen. She responded, "Star of Bethlehem." She then proceeded, without any prompting, to share that she had been the victim of rape several years ago. She stated that she thought she was "over it." I explained to her what was taking place: Star of Bethlehem was now healing another layer. Evidently, she was particularly sensitive. She was able to feel the further release of this profound and painful personal trauma.

I then asked if she would take some Rescue to ease her discomfort. She agreed, and I placed several drops in a glass of water. At this point I queried if there was a counselor present, since this young woman needed assistance to privately process her experience. I would need to temporarily stop the class and work through her crisis with her if there was no counselor available. To my relief, a counselor graciously stepped forward to help out with this crisis. The young woman left the room for fifteen minutes or so, Rescue Remedy in hand, and accompanied by the counselor. Upon returning, the young woman was again composed and able to resume participating.

Many individuals that I have counseled have chosen Star for similar reasons. They have also been victims of rape or incest. Yet, none of them has experienced the emotional intensification that this young woman at my seminar did. I repeat that this is a very rare occurrence. I have personally used Star for a bereavement issue and found it to bring great comfort and release of my grief.

HELPING OTHERS

As you work with Bach Flowers and personally experience the remarkable help available, you may find yourself wanting to help your loved ones. The more familiar you become with the flower essence indications, the easier it will be to assist others. In treating infants and young children, you will need to observe them and determine what negative emotional states are current. They may be unable to communicate these verbally. As a wrong selection of essence can do no harm, there is no need for concern about making an error. This is so encouraging to know, especially for new users who are uncertain with selection. The dosage is the same for children as it is for adults. The recommended maximum of seven flower essences, given four times daily, also applies to children.

I remind you not to give children the essences directly from the concentrate bottle due to the high alcohol content. Place the essences either in juice or other liquid, or prepare a personal dilution bottle. Don't be surprised when you find the reaction time in children to be quicker than with adults.

I remind you that pets and other animals also do exceptionally well with Bach Flowers. You will find that there are times when your pets, or any other animals that may be in your care, may suffer from stress, or experience emotional strain. Animals do experience emotions, as any pet owner will attest. Often, animals become ill at ease when major changes are taking place in their environment, such as a move, a new animal coming into the home, or perhaps the birth of a child, the loss of a familiar companion (human or animal), or even their human going through a major transition. Some animals that are adopted may have suffered abuse by a previous owner, and now cope with the effects of the trauma. The process of aging affects our pets as it does us, and they contend with illness and/or wounds from accidents or fights with other animals.

Just as the Bach Flowers restore balance to our energetic system, they are able to reinstate balance in our pets. To determine the appropriate essences for animals, imagine yourself in their situation. Ask yourself how you would feel under the same conditions. Your feelings, most likely, will be on target. When you are in doubt as to which specific essence to use, recall that Rescue is always helpful. I give my pets Rescue every day to maintain their general well-being.

The recommended dosage, and the limit of seven essences to be taken four times daily, applies to animals. Be aware that animals will refuse the drops from the concentrate because of the alcohol content. Therefore, it is best to administer the essences diluted in water. Place the drops in their drinking bowl or make them their very own dilution bottle. You may have several pets needing different essences. It is possible to mix the essences together in their common water bowl, or prepare a single dilution bottle. The animals will not react to the essences they don't need. The following case history is presented to facilitate your understanding of how flower essences are selected for animals.

Linda was given a puppy (which she named Hero) for her birthday. She already had two adult male cats, Crystal and Midnight. Initially, the cats did not appreciate the new addition to their family. This was no surprise, as there is always an adjustment period that takes place when a new pet comes into the home. Three-year-old Midnight had no trouble accepting Hero after the first several days. In fact, he considered him a new playmate. Seven-year-old Crystal, the dominant animal in the home, not only rejected the puppy, but would take swipes at him whenever the opportunity arose. This caused Hero to yelp in pain. Linda hoped that in the next week or two Crystal would come around to accepting the puppy as had Midnight.

It was not to be. A month had passed and the situation only worsened. Linda was now concerned that Crystal would badly injure the tiny puppy. Something had to be done. As Linda had been using the flower essences herself, she felt they might also be helpful with her pets. After she related the situation to me, the following flower essences were chosen.

Essences for Crystal
- Vine for his dominating nature, the "boss" animal
- Holly for his jealousy
- Cherry Plum for his aggressive, acting out behavior
- Walnut for transition, to help in adjusting to a new pet in the home
- Willow for his resentment
- Chestnut Bud for his failure to learn to stop his aggressive behavior

Essences for Hero
- Larch to boost his self-confidence
- Mimulus to ease his fear of Crystal
- Star to release the shock and trauma of Crystal's attack
- Walnut for transition, to help in adjusting to his new home

Linda reported that within less than a week Crystal was no longer attacking Hero. He would even let the puppy lick his ears! It would seem that by this act on Hero's part, he was no longer afraid of being hurt by the cat. Linda was no longer worried about Crystal harming Hero and peace once again reigned in their home.

Three months have now passed, and Crystal still behaves himself. Linda has not as yet discontinued the essences. She plans to do so in another month or two and has decided to continue to give Vine to Crystal, to keep his "Vine Personality" type in balance.

From the above illustration, you are able to see how animals can experience very similar negative emotional states as us (including feeling jealousy and resentment). Linda was certain that this was the case with Crystal. Whenever Linda played with the puppy, Crystal would also come over for some attention—which he wanted more, now that Hero was around. By imaginatively putting yourself in the animal's place, you can, as I've noted, get a sense of what is going on with your pet.

Don't forget your plants. Plants in distress respond beautifully to the flower essences. Try some Rescue in a vase of cut flowers to prolong their life. Rescue is also a life-saver for plants in shock from transplanting. Crab Apple is a great help with insect infestation.

When working with older children and adults, begin by explaining that the flower essences facilitate the release of difficult emotions they may be experiencing, and of personal issues that are concerning them. Have them then share what may be problematic in their lives. By listening to their words, you will be able to determine which essences are needed. Without doubt, you will hear the indications for the flower essences that they need.

Are they experiencing "fear" (Mimulus)? Do they lack "patience" (Impatiens)? Is "bitterness" or "resentment" being expressed (Willow)? Do they feel "taken advantage of" (Centaury)? Are they ridden with "guilt" (Pine)? Do they feel "hopeless" (Gorse)? You will hear words like these as they express their feelings to you. You may want to have paper and pen handy to jot down the key words they say. In this way, you can also be ready to repeat back what they have said in support of why you may suggest a particular essence.

It is imperative that you not be the one who makes the final selection for anyone you are helping. Consider yourself a guide, without forcing the issue. You may feel sure that they need a particular essence. But if they reject your suggestion, honor their personal healing process and their readiness to work on certain issues. Just as you may be in denial over some of your issues and are not ready to approach them as yet, others may also hesitate. And this is right and perfect. Be gentle and give them the same respect you would give yourself. Allow others to choose the flower essences that they are ready to work with and the issues they are ready to release. Remember, to begin any journey it is necessary to take that first step.

INTEGRITY WITH FLOWER ESSENCE USE

I am often asked whether flower essences can be given to others without their knowledge. My personal answer is no. It is only right that we have permission before offering help to another. Honesty is always the best policy. It would be best for all concerned that consent is given. I leave the final answer to this question to your own discretion, but remember, what goes around comes around.

There are, however, certain circumstances that do permit our administering the flower essences without consent, particularly to those who are unable to ask for our help. As parents and caregivers of our young children, we are charged with their care and empowered to help them in all possible ways. If we are guardians of individuals with cognitive handicaps who are unable to reason for themselves (those who are mentally retarded, the aged who suffer from Alzheimer's or dementia, or individuals diagnosed with mental illness), we are also obligated to assist with their care. And we may also step in with those individuals who are unconscious and unable to make decisions regarding their own care. To administer the flower essences to those who are unconscious, simply apply the essences to the pulse points and moisten their lips. Misting the room with a spray bottle containing appropriate essences is also helpful.

In the chapter that follows, you are given the opportunity to test your knowledge of the flower essence indications. This is offered to further your understanding, enhance your skill, and build your confidence with the selection process in your personal use and practice.

5.

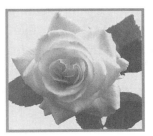

Practice Exercises in Selection

By presenting specific case studies which allow your practice of selection (with the answers available at the end of the chapter), you will have a model to refer to that facilitates your own use and practice with the Bach Flowers. As I have learned, it is always a boon to have such a reference to guide me along on any new path. I am confident that in a very short while, however, you no longer will need it. In the following exercises, case histories are offered for your consideration. As you read them, note which flower essences you would recommend to remedy the issues presented for that individual's situation. At the end of each case history, you will be given the specific number of essences that are indicated for that individual. Do your best in selecting the essences indicated in each case scenario. I've given you some assistance by highlighting the issues of each person which indicate his or her need for an essence. Please remember that these exercises are to help you, not to stress you out. Good luck.

CASE HISTORY #1

Kathy has begun her transition into menopause. She is a healthy and active woman, appearing younger than her fifty-two years of age. Yet, this life change brings up the fear of aging for her, as well as creating a loss of confidence in herself as a woman. She is concerned that she will no longer be sexually attractive to her husband. Aging had never been an issue for her until now. She is grieving over the loss of her youth, and feels bitter over her possible devaluation in a society that she believes puts youth on a pedestal.

Five flower essences are indicated for Kathy.

1.
2.
3.
4.
5.

CASE HISTORY #2

Janet is concerned over the recent change in behavior of her eight-year-old son, Brian. His teacher has called several times in the last two weeks, indicating that he has become disruptive in the classroom. He is fighting with his classmates, having temper outbursts, and is generally out of control. This surprises Janet. When Brian is at home he appears somewhat withdrawn and sad, not her usual, cheerful little boy. He has also begun to have frequent nightmares in the last week or so, waking up in terror. Janet is beginning to wonder if the pending divorce between her and Brian's father is now affecting their son. Is his recent change in behavior and the nightmares he is having the result of the loss he is experiencing? Brian's father moved out of their home a little over three weeks ago, and the whole family is now coping with major changes.

Four flower essences are indicated for Brian.

1.
2.
3.
4.

CASE HISTORY #3

Rita is an anxious woman in her mid-forties. She had developed diabetes some ten years ago, soon after her father's death. She has always felt guilty that she wasn't at the hospital when he died. This loss is still an issue for her. She never had the chance to say good-bye. Rita is also an overly anxious mother. She tends to worry a great deal over her children, always concerned for their welfare and safety. She is also plagued by constant anxiety and apprehension, unsure where this fear is coming from.

Four flower essences are indicated for Rita.

1.
2.
3.
4.

CASE HISTORY #4

Marci has just ended a seven-year relationship. This has become a difficult time of transition. She is grief-stricken over her loss. She is also blaming herself, feeling it was somehow her fault. Her self-confidence is all but gone, and she is sure that something must be lacking in her to have caused the break-up. Marci is now finding it hard to move on with her life, caught up in past memories, wishing she could turn back time. With her deep emotional trauma of loss, she now finds her energy totally dissipated.

Six flower essences are indicated for Marci.

1.

2.

3.

4.

5.

6.

CASE HISTORY #5

Russ' parents had just gotten divorced. He had been attending college away from home when the divorce took place. He would be graduating in a few months and was now faced with deciding which parent to live with. This was difficult for him as he loved both very much. Added to this issue was his grief over the loss of his family and the home where he grew up. He was finding it hard to adjust to this difficult transition, still longing for the way it used to be.

Four flower essences are indicated for Russ.

1.

2.

3.

4.

CASE HISTORY #6

Ann was in her eighth month of pregnancy and expecting twins. She was inexperienced as a mother. This was her first pregnancy, and she felt totally overwhelmed at the prospect of caring for two infants at once. She also found herself doubting her capabilities, certain she'd fail as a mother. As her time was fast approaching, Ann was now fearful of giving birth. Her doctor had advised that a cesarean section might be necessary. She could not get the thought of a possible operation off her mind. She was in the midst of an emotional crisis, unable to relax.

Five flower essences are indicated for Ann.

1.

2.

3.

4.

5.

CASE HISTORY #7

Sam, now in his early twenties, had a troubling childhood, with issues that have not as yet been resolved. At the age of seven, he had been diagnosed with learning disabilities. This had set the stage for the development of poor self-esteem and feelings of failure, which he is now dealing with. To cope with these deep-seated issues, Sam has become substance dependent to help ease his feelings of inner torment. Many times, while under the influence of alcohol, the rage he has been holding within explodes, his anger out of control. He also experiences bouts of depression, feeling hopeless with the circumstances of his life. In part, this has to do with a career he finds unfulfilling. Yet, he is afraid to make any changes, fearing his loss of security. He has now become resigned to the unhappy conditions of his life, feeling that there is nothing he can do to improve it.

Seven flower essences are indicated for Sam.

1.

2.

3.

4.

5.

6.

7.

CASE HISTORY #8

James is going through a very difficult time, feeling highly stressed with the circumstances taking place in his life. His elderly father suffers from Alzheimer's, and his mother is really not strong enough to care for him. Yet, she refuses to place him in a home. James is constantly worried about both his parents and their welfare. At the same time, he is the guardian of an aunt who is now in the hospital and in the process of dying. The doctors are ignoring her living will, refusing to cooperate, and James has had to seek legal counsel to ensure that his aunt's wishes will be honored. James is quite angry and resentful over this. Between concern for his parents and taking care of his aunt, he is totally overwhelmed by all his responsibilities.

Four flower essences are indicated for James.

1.
2.
3.
4.

CASE HISTORY #9

Elaine, a widow in her seventies, has always found it difficult in setting boundaries or standing up for herself, tending to serve others at her own expense. Regrettably, she has also allowed others to direct the course of her life as she is easily influenced by others. She is a shy and timid woman with many fears that have prevented her from living a more fulfilling life. Elaine also suffers from feelings of inferiority. Although she would like to make new friends (she has few), her low self-esteem limits her from doing so. Despite not being truly happy, she has accepted her life the way it is, lacking motivation to initiate any changes.

Five flower essences are indicated for Elaine.

1.
2.
3.
4.
5.

CASE HISTORY #10

Jeff had been diagnosed with cancer over six months ago, the news initially putting him into a state of shock and trauma. He immediately underwent radiation and chemotherapy, with his disease seemingly now under control. However, he finds himself not trusting his progress and fearful that the cancer will return. Although the malignancy has been destroyed, there remains a sense of his feeling unclean and contaminated. There are also feelings of anger and resentment over his disease. It just does not seem fair to him. He is only in his mid-thirties and feels that he has so much yet to accomplish in his life. His energy level is now quite low, depleted by his treatment and by his struggle to get well. He is not the type to give up easily, and he continues to bravely fight on. Yet, at times, he feels his situation is hopeless.

Seven flower essences are indicated for Jeff.

1.
2.
3.
4.
5.
6.
7.

ANSWER KEY

Case History #1

1. *Walnut* for Kathy's state of transition (menopause)
2. *Mimulus* for her fear of aging
3. *Larch* for her loss of self-confidence as a woman
4. *Star* for her grief over the loss of her youth
5. *Willow* for her resentment towards society

Case History #2

1. *Cherry Plum* for Brian's temper tantrums
2. *Star* for his grief over the divorce (shown by his withdrawal and sadness)
3. *Rock Rose* for his nightmares and terror
4. *Walnut* for his transition caused by divorce

Case History #3

1. *Pine* for Rita's guilt regarding her father
2. *Star* for her loss of her father
3. *Red Chestnut* for her overconcern for her children
4. *Aspen* for her anxiety and apprehension

Case History #4

1. *Walnut* for Marci's transition (ending a relationship)
2. *Star* for her grief over losing Jack
3. *Pine* for her guilt and self-blame
4. *Larch* for her loss of self-esteem
5. *Honeysuckle* for her dwelling in the past
6. *Olive* for her exhaustion over her emotional struggle

Case History #5

1. *Walnut* for Russ' transition caused by divorce
2. *Scleranthus* for his deciding which parent to live with
3. *Star* for his grief at losing home and family
4. *Honeysuckle* for his longing for the past

Case History #6

1. *Elm* for Ann's being overwhelmed by her new role as a mother of twins
2. *Larch* for her lack of confidence in her ability to adequately parent
3. *Mimulus* for her fear of childbirth
4. *White Chestnut* for her obsessing over the possibility of a c-section
5. *Rescue* for her emotional crisis and inability to relax

Case History #7

1. *Larch* for Sam's low self-esteem
2. *Agrimony* for his self-medication to repress his inner torment
3. *Cherry Plum* for his lack of control with alcohol and drugs and his violent temper
4. *Gorse* for his hopelessness over his life
5. *Wild Oat* for his discontent with his job
6. *Mimulus* for his fear that prevents his making a career change
7. *Wild Rose* for his resignation and inability to initiate positive changes in his life, thus remaining stuck where he is

Case History #8

1. *Rescue* for James' stress and anxiety over the crises playing out in his life
2. *Red Chestnut* for his deep concern for his parents and aunt
3. *Willow* for his resentment towards the doctors and their lack of cooperation
4. *Elm* for his being overwhelmed by great responsibilities towards his relatives

Case History #9

1. *Centaury* for Elaine's lack of boundaries and subservient attitude
2. *Walnut* for her being easily influenced by others and not living her own life
3. *Mimulus* for her timidity and fearful nature
4. *Larch* for her lack of self-confidence
5. *Wild Rose* for her resignation towards the circumstances of her life

Case History #10

1. *Star* for Jeff's shock and trauma when diagnosed with cancer
2. *Mimulus* for his fear of cancer ending his life
3. *Crab Apple* for his sense of contamination in having cancer
4. *Willow* for his resentment in contracting cancer, his sense of unfairness
5. *Olive* for his depletion of energy
6. *Oak* for his struggle and endurance
7. *Gorse* for his sense of hopelessness

I trust these exercises helped you, and built your confidence to select flower essences for specific, common issues and situations. If you should find yourself confused with, or doubting, any of the selections found in the Answer Key, you may want to review Chapter 3, A Review of The "39 Healers." The indications for all thirty-nine flower essences are thoroughly explored in that chapter. The more you work with the flower essences, the deeper your understanding of them, and your ease in remembering the indications for each, will become.

I have a strong sense that soon you will find yourself "hearing the essences speak to you" through the words that people use in conversation with you. Don't be surprised if you find you are typing the personalities of those you know well. Perhaps you now recognize mom personifying "Red Chestnut," "Chicory," or "Water Violet"? Is your dad seemingly an "Agrimony," "Rock Water," or "Vervain"? Is your best friend maybe a "Cerato," "Pine," or "Larch"? And is your boss possibly a "Beech," "Vine," or "Impatiens"?

With his flower essences, Dr. Bach has made it possible for us to understand our human nature better, and to make positive life changes.

We have completed Part One in our study of the Bach Flowers. The information thus far presented offers you a firm handle on traditional Bach Flower practice, and its use for yourself and others. Part Two helps you expand your use and practice of Dr. Bach's system of flower essences.

Part Two

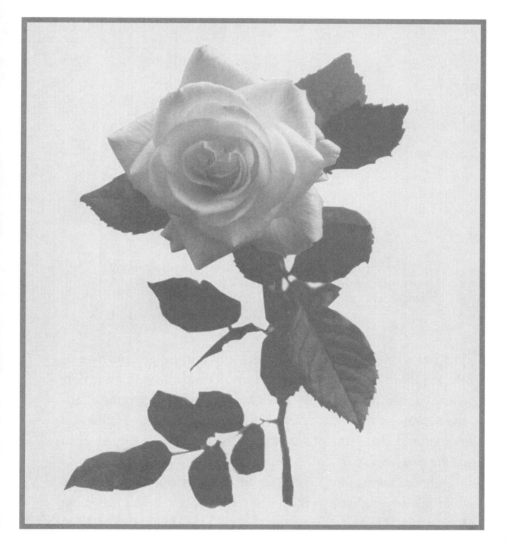

TRANSPERSONAL USE AND PRACTICE

6.

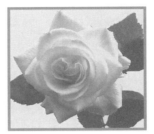

Affirmations

...Healing of the physical without the change in the mental
and spiritual aspects brings little real help to the individuals
in the end.

—*Edgar Cayce,* Reading 4016-1

We now explore additional support for your use and practice of
Bach Flower Therapy—affirmations. These enhance your personal healing process. Using affirmations will increase the effectiveness of your flower essence therapy. You will also achieve a
deeper and richer understanding of the positive quality in each
of the essences.

I have created thirty-eight inspiring affirmations that correlate
to each of the individual Bach Flower Essences. It was my intent
to capture the *positive potential*, or *virtue*, that each essence
embodies. Knowing their positive virtues, you can relate more
effectively on a conscious level to the energy that you are working
with, and empower your healing process. A brief explanation of
the technique of affirmations will help us begin.

We start with the understanding that we are primarily spiritual beings, in a body, and using a mind—a trinity of body,

mind, and spirit. When our personality is in alignment with our spiritual purpose, we are in harmony and experience health (wholeness). When this is not the case, we begin to suffer from dis-ease on subtle levels. Eventually, this imbalance filters down to the material level with the manifestation of physical disease. It is, therefore, crucial for each of us to become aware of the power of the mind. Our beliefs and thoughts have a great effect on our well-being on an energetic level. Dr. Bach based his system of healing on this premise. As the flower essences re-establish harmony to any negative emotional or mental states that are out of balance, then equilibrium, or homeostasis, is reinstated to our multidimensional system.

In Dr. Bach's understanding, disease is the result, an end product and final stage, of something much deeper. The true cause of any pathology originates above the physical plane, nearer to the mental. Illness is the result of a conflict between our spirit and personality. So long as these aspects of ourselves are in harmony, we have perfect health. It is only when discord arises between these aspects that the manifestation of disease is possible. Dr. Bach also held that illness is sent to us as a method of correction. We bring it entirely upon ourselves as the result of our own wrong doing and wrong thinking. Once we are able to recognize and then correct our fault(s), proceeding to live in harmony with the divine plan, disease will no longer be a part of our lives.

In our use of the Bach Flowers, we are beginning to consciously address the underlying disharmony that exits within us. We are choosing specific flower essences that relate to our emotional and mental distress. This awareness can be further increased as we learn to employ the technique of affirmations. In this modality we are using our mental bodies even more fully as we bring positive thoughts to consciousness. With these positive thoughts, we are setting the stage for our inner healer to be awakened, taking an active role in maintaining a healthy physical vehicle—the awesome body in which we live.

Be aware of the crucial role that our emotions play in the successful use of affirmations. It is imperative to allow ourselves to feel the power of what we are affirming, for our feeling nature (the emotional body) adds fuel to the fire. Without this element of deep feeling, our affirmations will fall flat. Our feelings hold the power of creation and manifestation. Godfrey Ray King, in his *Original Unveiled Mysteries*, tells us that the feeling activity of life is the most unguarded point of human consciousness. Our feelings become the cumulative energy by which thoughts become things. Thoughts without the backing of our emotions are powerless. The importance of guarding our feeling nature cannot be emphasized too strongly. The control of our emotions plays the most important part of anything in life. It maintains balance in the mind, health in the body, success and accomplishment in the affairs of the personal self of every one of us. As Godfrey Ray King emphasizes, "Thoughts can never become things until they are clothed with feeling."

As we work with affirmations, let us remember that as we create positive thoughts, we need to allow ourselves to feel the emotions related to these thoughts, as deeply and as powerfully as possible. We need to know that it is manifesting now, in the present, even though we cannot as yet see the results.

Simply put, an affirmation is a positive thought that we are creating. We then empower it with as much feeling as possible, to bring a positive outcome to what we desire. Our trust in what we are affirming is also crucial—that it is happening now. Know it is on its way to manifesting. As Dr. Wayne Dyer has said, "You'll see it when you believe it." Absolute faith and trust are the keys to manifestation.

Before anything can appear in the physical, it must first appear as an idea. The thought of anything is the first step in bringing it into form. The building of a house illustrates this. Before our house can become a physical reality, we must first think of, and then desire it. It initially appears as an idea in the mind. Once the idea has taken root in desire (emotion), the way is found (focus and intention) to make it a reality. Perhaps an architect is then hired to draw up the blueprints for our house. Soon the idea is on paper and is now visible. Once the right and perfect design has been established, the contractors are hired and the materials purchased. Within several months or so, the house has been built. What was once an idea in the mind alone, is now a physical, tangible, material reality with the application of our desire, focus, and intention.

Actually, we are always creating our reality, mostly unconsciously, with our positive or negative thoughts and emotions. As we become aware of this truth, we then are empowered to choose more wisely what we allow ourselves to think and to feel. We do have a choice in what we experience in our lives. Remember, *energy follows thought*. Whatever we choose to dwell on is manifested in our very lives. The more we are in the energy of fear, the more fear we attract. Conversely, the more we are in the energy of love, the more love we attract. Which would you rather have manifest in your life?

As beings with cognitive powers, we do have the choice to decide what we hold in our minds. When we are going through a difficult time, we can continue to concentrate on our misfortune, or we can choose to move through and past this, and allow our healing. This is especially true when we realize that all experiences that come to us are lessons—and that, in fact, we had agreed to take on these particular lessons before incarnating. We can choose to make the effort to grow from our experiences. Conscious use of affirmations is a tool that cultivates and promotes a positive state of mind.

In your use of affirmations with flower essences, you will discover that affirmations not only enhance their efficacy, but they can bring positive results much more rapidly in your healing process. The affirmations I have created are meant only as a guide for you. Perhaps at some point you may feel confident enough to create your own. I urge you to do so—you may find that you will relate even more strongly to your personal affirmations. As mentioned before, your feeling nature is a very important part of this process.

In your review of the affirmations that follow, have a pen and paper handy so that you may copy those that correlate to the flower essences you are presently using. Once you note the affirmations you are going to use, you will repeat each of these (preferably out loud if possible) three times whenever you take your flower essences. This repetition will help to anchor the affirmations into your subconscious mind. Privacy, and an attitude of reverence, are also important and will facilitate your success.

Depending on how many essences you are using, it may be too cumbersome to repeat each affirmation every time you are taking your essences. You may choose to work with a single affirmation each day, rotating through them all until you have completed the group. When this is done, repeat this process.

This is only a suggestion. Please work in whatever way is best for you. You are now ready to begin your personal empowerment of the flower essences you are taking. You will find that affirmations will facilitate a new awareness of, and cooperation with, the conscious changes you desire to bring about in your life.

Affirmations for the 38 Bach Flowers

Agrimony

I am aware of, in touch with, and accept my feelings and emotions. I allow myself to express them appropriately in all situations. I release myself from all hesitation to do so.

Aspen

I am safe and secure at all times. The light of God is my protection always. I trust in this power and release all fear of the unknown as I open to God's unfolding light.

Beech

I am tolerant towards everyone. I allow all to be who they are. I release all judgment towards others, with the awareness that we each do the best we are capable of.

Centaury

I allow my needs to be just as important as others' and can say no when their requests keep me from caring for myself. I release giving out of obligation as I honor Self. I give only when I feel so led.

Cerato

I trust my own judgment in decision making. I am aware of the still small voice within that is my constant source of wisdom. I release all self-doubt as I open to my inner guidance with confidence.

Cherry Plum

I am always in charge of all actions I take. I open to and accept the strength of the light within that guides me to right action. I release all fear of loss of control and know the power of self-control is mine.

Chestnut Bud

I learn from every experience that comes to me. I am open to and aware of the lesson in each experience that brings me growth. I release the need to repeat the same patterns again, and move on as I put into practice what I have learned.

Chicory

I give my love freely, without any demands. I am open to and accept the divine source of love within myself as my constant supply. Filled with this inner love, I release the need to manipulate or control others.

Clematis

I live in the present, grounded in the here and now. I accept the responsibility of my life and live it to the fullest. I release my need to escape, knowing this life is a divine gift.

Crab Apple

I am total perfection just as I am. I am as pure as the light that radiates within me, and accept my body in all ways as the perfect instrument for my life. I release all feelings of impurity or imperfection as I open to my inner radiance.

Elm

I am a highly capable and responsible person, able to handle all I need today. I have the skill to know what must be done now, and what can be left 'til tomorrow. I release concern of not accomplishing more than I can comfortably handle.

Gentian

I have faith in a Greater Wisdom working in all things. I accept delays and setbacks as part of this knowing. I release any despair, trusting that all is manifesting in perfect order and harmony.

Gorse

I look to the rainbow as a symbol of hope, as I open to and accept the promise of this within myself. I release all feelings of hopelessness to this eternal promise—after the rain, the rainbow.

Heather

I am interested in the welfare of others. I offer myself as a shoulder to lean on, knowing that the more I give, the more I shall receive. I release my needs of self interest and open to the empathy I hold within.

Holly

I feel the welling up of an all-encompassing love from deep within my being. I make peace with all past hurts as I am now able to let go. I forgive and release everything I feel has hurt me. As I love, so I am loved.

Honeysuckle

I choose to live in the present, no longer dwelling in past memories. I accept and look forward to today, to new experiences and surprises, feeling alive and vital. I release yesterday and say that today is the first day of my life.

Hornbeam

I am filled with inner vitality and feel refreshed in body, mind, and spirit. I open to and accept the Divine Light that flows through me, strengthening me as I release all fatigue.

Impatiens

I am filled with patience and easily go with the flow. I allow others to move at their own pace, knowing that we each have our own rhythm. I release the need to rush and hurry as I take time to smell the flowers.

Larch

I am in touch with my specialness and feel good about myself. I have self-worth and know that I can succeed at whatever I set out to do. I release my fear of failure, all feelings of self-doubt, as I move out in confidence.

Mimulus

Courage is mine as I am in touch with what has always been inside myself waiting to be freed. I open to and accept the cutting of old bonds of limitation. All fears are released to my new feelings of safety and security.

Mustard

My feelings of sadness are dissolved as the inner awareness of serenity now fills my being. I release all melancholy as I am open to the joy available from within.

Oak

My inner strength sustains me at all times. Yet I know when to endure and when to release and let go. I now allow myself to rest when there is need, and in doing so find I am renewed.

Olive

I am regenerating my inner vitality as I open to and am filled with a resurging energy that flows through me. I release all exhaustion as I am lovingly bathed in this healing light.

Pine

I am aware that I always do the best I am able, and in this awareness find satisfaction in all that I do. I release all regret and guilt of not being good enough and forgive myself, knowing that I am doing my best at all times.

Red Chestnut

I am filled with peace of mind concerning the welfare of those I love. I am aware that each is walking their own life path, as I am. I release all worry and fear regarding them in trust to a higher power.

Rock Rose

I am calm and serene in the face of all terror and panic, knowing I am in control. I open to and accept the courage that lies deep within me. Releasing my fears, I remain steadfast through all that appears a threat.

Rock Water

My inner convictions and ideals are a source of strength to me. Yet I am aware of the need for flexibility in living my life. I release and free myself from the chains of rigidity, and in doing so find inner freedom and new joy.

Scleranthus

I am filled with certainty as I weigh and balance all choices. I no longer vacillate between both ends, and with confidence make my decision. I am freed from all hesitation and self-doubt.

Star of Bethlehem

I am filled with the healing light that soothes all grief and loss. I open to and accept this gift of grace available from within. I release all sorrow, all trauma I have suffered, from my being. I am now restored and made whole.

Sweet Chestnut

My inner endurance rises up to fill me as I open to and accept this strength to go on. I am released from all feelings of anguish and despair, as the light from within breaks through this darkness and opens my heart to life.

Vervain

My inner gift of wisdom is to be shared only when asked. I use restraint in offering my opinions to others, knowing each is entitled to believe as they choose. I release the need to always be right and am filled with peace.

Vine

I am aware of my gift of leadership. I open to and accept this gift in humility, using my position of authority for the good of all. I lead gently and with love, and release my need to always dominate, as I listen to others' advice.

Walnut

I am aware that all new beginnings are a part of the wonderful adventure of life. I open to and accept these transitions as I break away from the past and all that binds me. In my release, I welcome the new in firm trust and faith.

Water Violet

I am aware that my gentleness, independence, and self-reliance are a source of strength to others. I willingly share my gifts in humility, as I release my need to detach from others as I hear the call to serve.

White Chestnut

My mind is now stilled as I open to the peace that lies at the core of my being. I open to and accept this tranquility, which, like a soft blanket, quiets all unwanted thoughts. I release all concerns and find peace of mind.

Wild Oat

From deep within me, my purpose rises clear. I accept and open to this inner knowing that leads me to my life's work. I release uncertainty and feelings of unfulfillment as I trust this divine guidance.

Wild Rose

Life is taking on new meaning for me. I am in touch with the excitement and joy it has to offer. It is in my power to choose this, and I do so now. I release my indifference to what has been and make the effort to live anew.

Willow

I accept and am open to personal responsibility for my life. It is time to move past blaming others for my problems, as I realize each did the best they could. I move into forgiveness and release all resentment from my heart.

I would like to offer one more suggestion in your work with affirmations. It would be very helpful to create your personal affirmation audiotape by recording the ones you are using. Record each affirmation three times slowly, and with as much feeling as possible. Go on until all your selections are recorded. Your personal affirmation tape can be played every morning, as you get dressed, to set a positive tone for the day. Played again at night, as you are going to sleep, it reinforces the positive messages you are placing into your subconscious mind. Listening to the sound of your own voice can impress the subconscious even more deeply. When you change your flower essences (as most of us do as we continue to change and grow), simply record the next group of affirmations onto a new tape. Know that you are involved in very special work here. You are consciously taking your power back in facilitating your own well-being.

The affirmations presented in the chapter have been excerpted from my audio program, *Affirmations—Enhancing Bach Flower Therapy.* For those who would like to have all thirty-eight affirmations already recorded and ready to work with, please see the Resource section for information on ordering your personal copy.

In the chapter that follows you are shown how to apply information from your natal chart in your use of flower essences. The astrological birth chart is a modality that sheds light on the personality characteristics with which we are born. The Bach Flowers bring harmony to our negative personality traits; by examining our birth chart we are given another avenue towards discovering the aspects of our personality that are in need of balance. I have written this chapter for students of astrology as well as novices, to make this information available for all to use. I trust you will find what is presented valuable.

7.

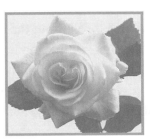

An Astrological Approach

Ever consider the Universe as One Living Being, with one material substance and one Spirit. Contemplate the fundamental causes, stripped of all disguise. Consider well the nature of things, distinguishing between matter, cause, and purpose.

—Marcus Aurelius

While we have no empirical means of measuring the emanations of the planets and stars, it appears that on some non-definable level they affect all of life to some degree. There is a unity underlying everything in existence, although this is not always apparent.

Since antiquity it has been observed that the position of the planets and stars seems to play a role in the happenings here on earth. From these early observations, astrology was born. When we are able to calculate the exact planetary picture in the heavens at the time, place, and date of an individual's birth, there appears to be a strong correlation between the energy of these planets and that of the individual. Our personality is colored by the energy pattern present in the sky at the moment of our first breath. It is as though we have "breathed in" this energy or vibratory pattern, which then proceeds to influence our development along certain lines throughout the course of our life.

Depending upon the signs of the zodiac the planets are moving through, as well as their aspect relationship to one another, an astute astrologer is able to define the basic personality characteristics of an individual. He or she then views the astrological chart as a map or guide which indicates a person's life pattern. Most of us are familiar with our Sun sign, which is the sign of the zodiac that the Sun was passing through on the day and month when we were born. However, this is not the complete picture of our natal energies. It is also necessary to know the signs of all the planets, including Mercury, Venus, Mars, Jupiter, Saturn, Uranus, Neptune, Pluto, and of course, the Moon, in their concurrent passage with the Sun through the zodiac.

Just as our Sun sign affects our basic ego drive and direction in life, each of the other known planets and signs at the time of our birth contributes to our many-faceted personality. The Moon sign symbolizes habit patterns from the past, and, most importantly, our emotional nature. Mercury's sign shows our mode of thinking and style of communication, while Venus' indicates our response to love, our values, and social graces. Mars' sign characterizes our energy drive and sexual expression, and Jupiter's indicates our societal values and expansiveness. Saturn's denotes where our duties and responsibilities lie, setting our boundaries, and is our cosmic teacher. Uranus' urges us on to freedom or to chaos, and Neptune's to inspiration or to delusion. Pluto's placement brings, whether we cooperate with it or not, the opportunity of purification and transformation in the eternal process of evolving to higher awareness.

We are given a clearer understanding of who we are and why we function as we do, when our own unique planetary picture can be ascertained. The natal chart is the puzzle, and the planets and their signs are the pieces we put together in discovering the mystery of self. Using the knowledge of astrology, we are better equipped to comprehend the nature of our present life. We are also better able to cope constructively with the lessons we have chosen to work through in this incarnation—which are delineated in our personal birth chart. With astrological insight, we come face-to-face with our life's path; that insight is also a tool by which we can better understand our soul's purpose.

Astrology is an invaluable tool for healing. The natal chart is a powerful description of positive and negative personality characteristics. If we are aware of these, we can change them—if we so choose. The Bach Flowers also correspond to our personality traits, and are compatible with astrology. The natal chart can be used as a strong indicator for the essences which are most suitable for an individual.

When I began my study of the flower essences and got to know their indications well, I found myself correlating different people in my life to the essence types. I remember how, as an astrologer, I could match astrological energies with individuals, before I knew their charts. As I began to study the Bach Flowers, I saw that the flower essence indications related very strongly to the archetypal energies of the twelve signs of the zodiac. They also correlated to the challenging aspects between planets in the birth chart.

Challenging aspects are determined by certain mathematical relationships between any two planets, at a particular moment in space and time, in their transit through the zodiac. Thus, the angle between two planets, as viewed in the three-hundred-and-sixty-degree circle of the zodiac, establishes an "aspect." Aspects are considered easy, when the energy between two planets is compatible, harmonious, and easily accessed by an individual. An aspect is considered challenging when the energy between two planets is incompatible, discordant, and causes a conflict within the individual as to how these conflicting energies are accessed.

To illustrate, when Mars and Saturn are in easy aspect, such as the trine, an individual is able to use his energy drive (Mars) positively—he succeeds in accomplishing his goals (Saturn) in a responsible, productive manner. There is a cooperative flow between how he takes action and the success of that action. Conversely, when Mars and Saturn are in a challenging aspect, such as the square, a person finds conflict and frustration in using his energy drive (Mars) to successfully accomplish the achievement of his goals (Saturn). It feels like he has one foot on the gas pedal and the other on the brake.

Dr. Bach originally developed only twelve flower essences. Soon after, he went on to develop the remaining twenty-six, calling them "helper" essences. As Dr. Bach had a deep metaphysical background, was it possible that the initial twelve essences were meant to correlate with the twelve signs of the zodiac on some level? And had he originally felt that only twelve essences were to be discovered?

There seems to be more than a hint of this (and of his knowledge of astrology) in an article written by Dr. Bach at Epsom, in 1933, and originally published in the *Naturopathic Journal*. Julian Bernard reprinted this article in his excellent book, *Collective Writings of Edward Bach*. In his article, entitled "Twelve Healers," Bach stated unequivocally that there are twelve personality types, with a positive and negative side to each. These twelve personality types are indicated by the sign the Moon is in at the time of an individual's birth. He also suggested that the study of the natal Moon sign will give us our personality type, point out our work to be done in this life, and indicate the flower essence that correlates to our personality type and assists us in that work.

In astrological symbology, the Moon reflects our emotional nature. Dr. Bach correlated personality types with natal Moon signs, and stated that these Moon signs influence and define our personality. Finding one's type essence can be very perplexing, but Dr. Bach has made this discovery easier, by giving us a remarkable guide.

In "Twelve Healers," Dr. Bach stated that healers basically deal with the negative side of the twelve personality types. The secret of life is to be true to our personality and not to allow interference from outside influences. Bach felt that astrologers put too much emphasis on the planets. If we can hold our personality and be true to ourselves, we need not fear any planetary or other outside influence. Our particular personality type essence (defined by one of the zodiac's twelve possible natal Moon signs) would assist us with this.

Dr. Bach also stated that it is only in our earlier stages of evolution that we are directly influenced by the planets. Once we develop love—the love of humanity—we are freed from our stars, from our fate, and free to steer our own ship. Dr. Bach noted that, with his original twelve essences, it was simple to prescribe accurately, and to help patients understand the reason for their disharmony and their disease. The essences teach them that they may be in tune with their souls, thereby restoring their mental and physical health.

Towards the end of his life, upon completing the development of his flower essences, Dr. Bach burned many of his papers. Despite the horrified cries of his assistants, he explained that he desired to eliminate any confusion with his previous writings in the interest of keeping his system as clear and simple as possible, for all to use. Apparently, Dr. Bach deleted information regarding astrology and the flower essences. There is no other information in any of the literature I've researched, regarding which of the twelve original essences specifically related to each of the possible twelve natal Moon signs of the zodiac. In his medical practice, Dr. Bach did treat his patients' personality, character, and mood. From his observations came what he termed the "Twelve Outstanding States of Mind."

DR. BACH'S TWELVE STATES OF MIND

1. Fear	7. Overconcern
2. Terror	8. Weakness
3. Mental Torture/Worry	9. Self-distrust
4. Indecision	10. Impatience
5. Indifference/Boredom	11. Overenthusiasm
6. Doubt/Discouragement	12. Pride/Aloofness

These are personality weaknesses that are to be overcome as we evolve. Dr. Bach's Twelve States of Mind correspond to the original Twelve Healers (his first twelve essences). These Twelve Healers, in turn, correspond to each of the zodiac's twelve possible natal Moon signs. The correlations in the following table are derived from my study and practice of astrology, and of Bach Flowers, over many years.

CORRELATIONS BETWEEN THE 12 STATES OF MIND/12 TYPE ESSENCES/12 NATAL MOON SIGNS

State of Mind	Type Essence	Natal Moon Sign
1. Impatience	Impatiens	Aries
2. Doubt/Discouragement	Gentian	Taurus
3. Self-distrust	Cerato	Gemini
4. Indifference/Boredom	Clematis	Cancer
5. Overenthusiasm	Vervain	Leo
6. Weakness	Centaury	Virgo
7. Indecision	Scleranthus	Libra
8. Overconcern	Chicory	Scorpio
9. Mental Torture/Worry	Agrimony	Sagittarius

10. Fear	Mimulus	Capricorn
11. Pride/Aloofness	Water Violet	Aquarius
12. Terror	Rock Rose	Pisces

We now examine these correlations more deeply, going through each of the possible twelve Moon signs, the states of mind related to these, and the type essence indicated for overcoming inherent weaknesses of your natal Moon sign. We will review only the negative manifestations of the Moon signs, as these are the qualities that are in need of balance. Of course, each sign has a positive quality as well. To ascertain your natal Moon sign for your type essence you will need your natal chart.

MOON SIGNS AND THE CORRELATING PERSONALITY TYPE ESSENCES

Aries Moon

Individuals with an Aries Moon are impulsive, known to take action before thinking first. The sign of the Ram is their symbol, and these individuals don't hesitate to butt heads. They also tend towards impatience, wanting what they want when they want it. Because they are too spontaneous in spirit, they are not tactful, and often hurt others' feelings by speaking without thinking first. They may not understand the needs of others, and feel their needs should be considered first. Their turbulent emotions are usually on the surface, and they tend to have temper outbursts of the moment. They feel restless and have difficulty completing what has been started, for they feel driven to move on to the next challenge. The flower essence *Impatiens* is the type essence for this Moon sign, bringing patience and a sense of gentleness towards others. This also facilitates their being able to relax and take the time to smell the flowers.

Taurus Moon

Individuals with a Taurus Moon can be prone to inertia. They are gentle souls easily discouraged by the ups and downs and twists and turns that are a normal part of life. In order to feel safe, these people always seek security, on all levels. They have a tendency towards procrastination. They feel "why bother?" when their efforts prove futile, and this feeling causes a loss of faith to take root. At the start, they expect that whatever they desire should easily come to them. When it doesn't, they give up and become complacent—impossible to move, just like the Bull, their symbol. The flower essence *Gentian* is the type essence for this Moon sign, bringing faith in the implicit order of the universe, that there are reasons for setbacks and delays. Despair is released, dispelling all inertia, thus allowing the flow of movement once again.

Gemini Moon

Individuals with a Gemini Moon are at the mercy of their highly active minds—a constant barrage of ideas and thoughts leaves them exhausted. In their search for truth, there is a restlessness that scatters their energy. In their longing for knowledge, they often feel the need to go to others, for they don't trust their own intuition. Their lack of self-confidence in making decisions, and confusion caused by changing feelings, makes them appear as though they are two people in one, reflecting their symbol, the Twins. The feelings caused by their mental self-doubt often create states of deep anxiety and nervous tension. The flower essence *Cerato* is the type essence for this Moon sign, and it instills a sense of confidence in personal intuition. Uncertainty is released, allowing anxiety and nervous tension to dissipate. In their unending quest for knowledge, they now look within, rather than to others, for the answers.

Cancer Moon

Individuals with a Cancer Moon are extraordinarily sensitive, self-absorbed, and introverted people, like the Crab which symbolizes this sign. The imagination and intuition are highly developed, allowing them to pull into their "shell." They are easily absorbed in a world of their own making. Like the ever-changing phases of the Moon (the planet that rules this sign), these individuals are caught in the ebb and flow of their constantly shifting emotions, which are in turn affected by the environment around them. To protect themselves against their super-sensitive feeling nature, they often need to retreat. The flower essence *Clematis* is the type essence for this Moon sign, enabling these individuals to come out of their shell, to be in the present moment, to take part in life. This essence helps them put their incredible imagination to practical use, and overcome their tendency to get lost in daydreams and let life silently slip by. The meaning and purpose of their very being is realized as they begin to use their special gifts and talents.

Leo Moon

Individuals with a Leo Moon have a deep need to be noticed. As the Sun (which rules this sign) is the center of our solar system, these individuals want to be the center of attention in the lives of others—at home, in social situations, or at work. A sense of authority is inherent, as it is in their symbol, the Lion, king of the jungle. Their underlying desire for power, and need always to be right, make it almost impossible for anyone else to disagree with them. They must have the last word. With their strong feeling nature, they tend to become overenthusiastic about their beliefs. They are usually very strong and forceful personalities. The flower essence *Vervain* is the type essence for this Moon sign, bringing the wisdom of restraint as well as flexibility to these individuals. Their egocentricity is tempered, their natural leadership qualities are now appreciated and sought after, and they are an inspiration to all those they meet.

Virgo Moon

Individuals with a Virgo Moon have a strong desire to serve others, as exemplified by their symbol of the Virgin, the servant of the zodiac. Often this service is regrettably at their own expense. They are unable to create appropriate boundaries between themselves and other people and find it difficult to refuse any request made of them. There is a reserved and quiet air about them, a meekness to their manner, that prevents them from appropriately asserting themselves when necessary. Thus, they find themselves easily taken advantage of by others. In their extreme willingness to serve, they may neglect their own mission in life. The flower essence *Centaury* is the type essence for this Moon sign, balancing service to others with the ability to care for self. Their weakened or nonexistent boundaries are strengthened, as is their personal sense of purpose, with the understanding of authentic service to those truly in need.

Libra Moon

Individuals with a Libra Moon are beset by indecisiveness and vacillation, first swinging one way and then the other. They are always in a quandary and never quite sure if their choice is correct. Their sign is fittingly symbolized by the Scales. They are plagued by self-doubt, yet keep this to themselves and rarely ask others for help. The flower essence *Scleranthus* is the type essence for this Moon sign, instilling a sense of confidence in their ability to make decisions, and removing their tendency to vacillate back and forth and agonize over their choices.

Scorpio Moon

Individuals with a Scorpio Moon are known to have strong and deep emotions, to the point of brooding. They tend to be possessive with those they are close to, and to demand a great deal in relationships. Their feelings are easily hurt, especially when ignored. This tends to bring on bouts of moodiness. They have a dominating nature with a need for control. They feel they know what is best for others, and they are willing to manipulate to get what they desire. Like their symbol, the Scorpion, they would rather destroy themselves than give up. The flower essence *Chicory* is the type essence for this Moon sign, opening these individuals to the deep selfless love within that no longer makes demands of others, but freely gives of itself. The need for controlling others is released, and their possessive nature is no longer a burden to them or those they love.

Sagittarius Moon

Individuals with a Sagittarius Moon are often cheerful, friendly people with no one suspecting the torment hidden beneath the face they present to the world. They usually have many acquaintances, yet few close friends. There is a great restlessness inherent in them, demonstrated by their need to be constantly on the go—like the Centaur that is their symbol. These are the gamblers and adventurers of life, and they tend to take things to excess in all that they do. The flower essence *Agrimony* is the type essence for this Moon sign, soothing their restless nature and allowing them to be in touch with, and to heal, their inner torments. No longer do they need to run from themselves, or continue with the meaningless distractions of the past.

Capricorn Moon

Individuals with a Capricorn Moon are highly conservative, appear somewhat rigid and controlled in manner, and feel a deep need for approval by others. Insecurity is a major issue for this individual. There is a striving for achievement, driven by the fear of not being successful, not being seen as important and powerful. Their security lies in authority. Fear is the driving force behind these individuals—fear of failure in not achieving their lofty goals, and, even worse, fear of rejection. Appropriately, their symbol is the Mountain Goat, ever striving to climb that mountain. The flower essence *Mimulus* is the type essence for this Moon sign, bringing release to the many fears that have crystallized their feeling nature, instilling courage to be themselves without the need to prove anything to anyone else.

Aquarius Moon

Individuals with an Aquarius Moon tend to be cool and aloof, with a rigid and limited feeling nature, and a strong need for freedom and independence in relationships. Although they are good friends, they shun intimacy. While each of them is an "original" in personality, there is a sense of pride and possibly of superiority in their uniqueness, giving them an air of detachment. Their symbol, the Water Bearer, indicates the many gifts they have to share with humanity—once they learn humility. The flower essence *Water Violet* is the type essence for this Moon sign, allowing a melting of the cold veneer that keeps others at arm's length, and relieving the feeling of need for isolation. With a new willingness to share themselves honestly and openly, the sense of superiority is washed away in their realization that everyone is truly special.

Pisces Moon

Individuals with a Pisces Moon are extremely sensitive to the negative vibrations from others, feeling others' pain as if it were their own, many times suffering deeply from all the misfortune they perceive. With this placement, there is a divine discontent that nothing in this world will take away, for these people recognize on an inner level that the material world is only an illusion. Because they deeply long for another world they can only sense, living in the body is almost more than they can bear. Their symbol is the Fish. Two are tied together, swimming in different directions—one earth-bound and the other heaven-bound. Subtly pulled in two directions, the emotional nature is delicate and impressionable, rendering these people nervous, unstable, and reactive in personality. The flower essence *Rock Rose* is the type essence for this Moon sign, calming the deep inner terror of harsh material reality, and establishing firm standing for their sensitive and susceptible nature, in the midst of all worldly turmoil.

ESSENCES FOR CHALLENGING NATAL PLANETARY ASPECTS

We will now explore the Bach Flower Essences that would be indicated for each of the planets when involved in challenging aspects. (In the language of astrology, the Sun and Moon are termed "planets" for the sake of simplicity.) By no means is this an exhaustive study. It is meant as a generalized overview only, and may seem an oversimplification of astrological material. However, in the interest of learning and being able to make use of this information, this broad analysis gives us a place to start.

Astrology offers a powerful approach to flower essence selection, although this technique may not be as "simple" as the traditional approach that Dr. Bach left for the masses. I will present astrology clearly and simply, so that it can be used in flower essence selection even if you have no prior astrological expertise.

It is important to look at the hard or challenging aspects between natal planets. These include the square, where two planets' energies are in conflict, causing a struggle in their use, and indicated by a ninety-degree angle; the opposition, where two planets' energies are opposed, calling for the need to balance the polarities, and indicated by their being on opposite sides of the zodiac, one hundred and eighty degrees apart; and certain conjunctions involving the outer planets (Saturn, Uranus, Neptune, and Pluto), where two planets are transiting side by side, within ten degrees of one another, vying for domination

(See Figures 1, 2, 3 on the following pages). These challenging aspects appear to be the possible negative planetary influences (outside forces) that Dr. Bach alluded to. It would seem that the other twenty-six helper essences were then developed with these planetary energies in mind, to assist in freeing us from their adverse effects.

Challenging Aspects to the Moon

With an afflicted Moon, the following issues may be experienced: coping with insecurities (Mimulus); overdependency (Centaury); emotional loss of control, overindulgence with food, drugs, or alcohol (Cherry Plum); living in the past (Honeysuckle); an overconcern for loved ones (Red Chestnut); overinvolvement with loved ones and a need to manipulate and control their affairs (Chicory); the inability to nurture self or others (Centaury, Rock Water, Water Violet, Holly); holding on to past hurts (Willow); an extreme sensitivity to the environment (Walnut); escapist tendencies (Clematis).

Challenging Aspects to the Sun

With an afflicted Sun, the following issues may be experienced: excessive demands for attention (Chicory); egocentric (Vervain); controlling (Vine); poor self-esteem (Larch); timid and fearful (Mimulus); a lack of ego boundaries (Centaury); self-effacing (Pine); self-involved (Heather); selfish and demanding (Chicory); pride and vanity (Water Violet); jealous and possessive (Holly); overstriving (Oak); uncertain as to direction in life (Wild Oat).

Challenging Aspects to Mercury

With an afflicted Mercury, the following issues may be experienced: a restless mind, and/or obsessive thinking (White Chestnut); mental exhaustion leading to boredom (Hornbeam); an inability to concentrate (Clematis); an inability to make decisions (Cerato, Scleranthus); a lack of perception, often

CONJUNCTION
Figure 1

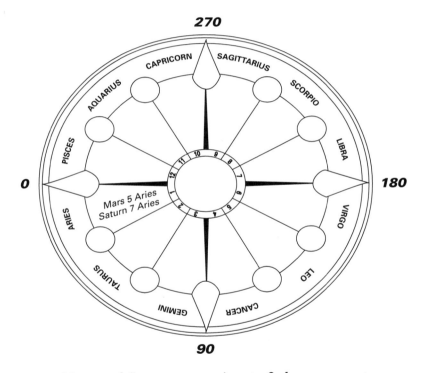

*Mars and Saturn are conjunct—2 degrees apart.
A conjunction is exact when planets are at the
same degree in the same sign. However, a 10
degree orb is allowed.*

SQUARE
Figure 2

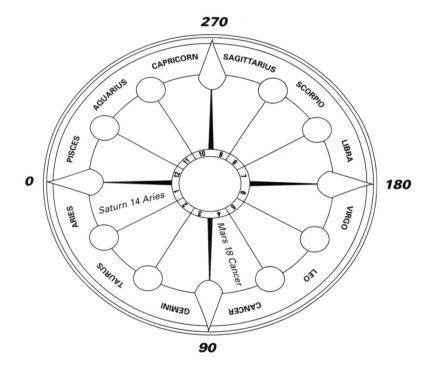

Mars and Saturn are square—94 degrees apart. A square is exact when planets are 90 degrees apart. However, there is an orb of 10 degrees on either side, beginning at 80 degrees and ending at 100 degrees.

OPPOSITION
Figure 3

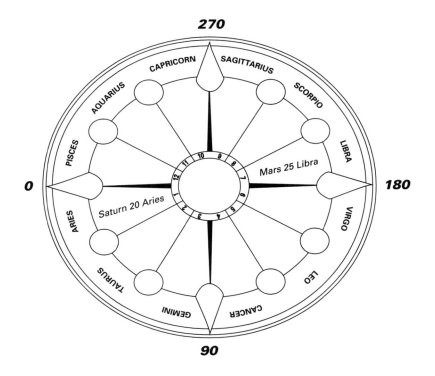

Mars and Saturn in opposition—185 degrees apart. An opposition is exact when planets are 180 degrees apart. However, there is an orb of 10 degrees on either side, beginning at 170 degrees and ending at 190 degrees.

repeating the same mistakes (Chestnut Bud); judgmental and intolerant (Beech); self-involved (Heather); a lack of confidence in ability to communicate or to learn, feeling inept (Larch); a need to proselytize (Vervain); a rigid and inflexible mindset (Vine, and possibly Rock Water with regard to one's personal ideals).

Challenging Aspects to Venus

With an afflicted Venus, the following issues may be experienced: a constant need for love and approval, with a weakening of personal boundaries (co-dependency) (Centaury); the inability to confront others (Agrimony); procrastination, and also easily discouraged (Gentian); fear of intimacy (Mimulus); obsession with personal appearance and/or dissatisfaction with the physical body (Crab Apple); self-involved (Heather), aloof and detached (Water Violet); vain and self-indulgent, possessive and jealous (Holly); manipulative and controlling in love (Chicory); indecisive (Scleranthus); easily deceived in love (Clematis).

Challenging Aspects to Mars

With an afflicted Mars, the following issues may be experienced: possessing a volatile temper and risk taking (Cherry Plum); easily frustrated, impatient, and tense (Impatiens); repression of anger (Agrimony); lack of initiative (Wild Rose, Gentian, Larch); competitive nature to the extreme (Vervain); aggressive or dominating (Vine); overdriven with mismanagement of energy (Oak, Vervain); manipulative and controlling (Chicory); deep inner rage, suspicion, and jealousy (Holly); fear of asserting self (Mimulus); overwhelmed by taking on too much (Elm); chronic fatigue (Olive); repeated misuse of energy (Chestnut Bud).

Challenging Aspects to Jupiter

With an afflicted Jupiter, the following issues may be experienced: arrogance (Vervain); judgmental nature (Beech); foolhardy (Cherry Plum); rigid and inflexible regarding new ideas (Vine, Vervain, or possibly Rock Water); being overwhelmed by taking on too much (Elm).

Challenging Aspects to Saturn

With an afflicted Saturn, the following issues may be experienced: perfectionist (Pine); rigid and controlling, demanding authority (Vine); fear of failure (Mimulus); easily gives up for lack of self-confidence (Larch); hypercritical (Beech); workaholic (Oak); melancholia (Mustard, and Gorse for hopelessness); apathy and resignation (Wild Rose); a hardness of heart (Holly).

Challenging Aspects to Uranus

With an afflicted Uranus, the following issues may be experienced: rebellion and non-conformity (Cherry Plum); aloof and independent to the extreme (Water Violet); a law unto themselves (Vine); rigid and inflexible ideals (Rock Water); a need to break with the past and from the influences of others (Walnut); the fear of their own uniqueness and expression of individuality (Mimulus); the need to always be right (Vervain, Vine).

Challenging Aspects to Neptune

With an afflicted Neptune, the following issues may be experienced: caught up in illusion (the rose-colored glasses syndrome), escapism, being self-deceptive or deceived (Clematis); self-sacrificing and easily taken advantage of (the saviors or martyrs), diffuse boundaries (Centaury); an addiction to drugs and alcohol to repress their oversensitivity to worldly pain and sorrow (Agrimony, Cherry Plum, Chestnut Bud); easily influenced by others (Walnut); anxiety attacks, pervasive feelings of foreboding

(Aspen); nervous, unstable, reactive personalities (existential terror) (Rock Rose).

Challenging Aspects to Pluto

With an afflicted Pluto, the following issues may be experienced: obsessive compulsive behavior and thoughts (Cherry Plum, White Chestnut); possessive, demanding, and manipulative (Chicory); a lack of trust bordering on paranoia at times, jealous, vengeful (Holly); domination over others (Vine); emotional intensity (Vervain); struggles on and endures at all costs (Oak); bitter and resentful (Willow); a tendency towards separateness and isolation (Water Violet); denial or repression of feelings (Agrimony).

A CONSIDERATION OF SATURN'S SIGN

Astrologers call Saturn "The Lord of Karma." The sign that Saturn occupied at our birth indicates inherent weaknesses in our personality. We have chosen to work through those weaknesses in this life. The appropriate Bach Flower Essence can help you with these issues. Consult the table on page 180; find the astrological sign that Saturn occupies in your natal chart, and read across to find the appropriate flower essence. Use that flower essence to enhance your personal growth. For example, if Saturn was in Aries at your birth, you would use Impatiens; if Saturn was in Cancer, Clematis is indicated.

A CONSIDERATION OF TRANSITS

A transit is the position of a planet in the zodiac at a specific moment in time. At the time of this writing, the planet Pluto is transiting (moving through) the zodiac sign of Sagittarius. There are thirty degrees in each sign, and Pluto is at the seventh degree of Sagittarius. Pluto, being so far out from the Earth, takes two hundred and forty-eight years to transit all twelve signs of the zodiac. Thus, in an individual's lifetime, it might move through no more than five or six signs.

Jupiter is much closer to the Earth, transiting through one sign in only a year. Thus, every twelve years it has transited all twelve signs. Each of the other planets, including the Sun and Moon, also transit at their own particular speed, depending on how close or far their position is in relation to the Earth.

Astrologers are able to determine the planetary transits by using an ephemeris. This is a book which logs the positions of all the planets in their movement through the heavens. My ephemeris has these placements calculated from the year 1900 through 2000. When I want to check the current transits of the planets, I simply locate the year, month, and day, as I did with Pluto.

Astrologers are always mindful of transits, as these transiting planetary energies activate the natal planets in an individual's horoscope (birth chart). To illustrate, let us use Pluto's current position of seven degrees Sagittarius. Pluto's emanations will affect any natal planet at the seventh degree. Depending on the aspect, the effect will be lesser or greater. The most intense aspects are the challenging ones—the conjunction, square, and opposition.

Those interested in taking the correlation between astrology and the Bach Flowers further may want to look at the current transits of the outer planets (Saturn, Uranus, Neptune, and Pluto). Astrologers pay particular attention to these, as the impact of their energies is of longer duration and, more profoundly life-changing.

If you undergo any transits that are activating natal planets in your birth chart, you will very likely experience some stress. By discovering the flower essences that correlate to any major transits taking place in your life, you will find the Bach Flowers to be of great assistance in coping with these major astrological cycles.

We will now explore the outer planet transits to the personal planets (Sun, Moon, Mercury, Venus, and Mars) in our natal chart, correlating this planetary movement with the flower essences that may be helpful during these change-producing times. Again, please note that generalizations are presented. No one will experience the same transits identically. We are all unique and individual. However, what is presented will give you an idea of the basic energies of each of the planetary transits and the lessons they bring to us.

SATURN TRANSITS

Saturn symbolizes maturity and responsibility, structure and form, and setting our boundaries—our limits. Saturn is also the "cosmic teacher," testing how far we have come in our development. If we have shirked our responsibilities, our duties, there will be a price to pay with Saturn's transits to our personal planets. Issues of self-worth and personal authority lie at the heart of Saturn's lessons.

Essences for Saturn Transiting the Sun

When under the "hard" (challenging) transits by Saturn to our natal Sun, we live in a time of self-appraisal, as the Sun symbolizes our sense of self. We look at who we are and what we have to offer the world. We may take a second look at our job or career and may decide that changes are needed (Wild Oat). This is generally a period of some new responsibility. If we haven't prepared well, it may be a difficult time. We may experience fear at the thought of a change (Mimulus), or feel overwhelmed by the added responsibility (Elm). We may also feel a sense of restriction or limitation—things seem stuck, bringing on frustration and impatience (Impatiens). Depression may also be a part of this experience, especially if we now find we're in a job or career that is not suited to us and we find unfulfilling (Gorse, Wild Oat). Setbacks and delays are common, with growing feelings of discouragement (Gentian). Fatigue is often an issue with all the stress being experienced (either Hornbeam or Olive, depending on the depth of exhaustion). Our self-esteem may be adversely affected (Larch). Resentment may creep in towards others we feel are holding us back or causing us problems (Willow). We may find ourselves working harder than ever, keeping our nose to the grindstone, and being too hard on ourselves (Oak).

Essences for Saturn Transiting the Moon

When under the hard transits by Saturn to our natal Moon, we live through a depressing time. The Moon symbolizes our feeling nature, and this is now under examination. Are our emotional needs being met? Probably not, right now. The need for affection is stronger at this time, and if we are not receiving what we need, depression may set in (Gorse) as well as a fear of being unlovable or unworthy (Mimulus, Larch). Resentment may also be experienced in this situation (Willow). There may also be a sense of emotional loss (and sometimes we do lose someone) (Star of Bethlehem). We also become more aware of our bodies. Do we need to lose some extra pounds? Is it time to start an exercise routine, and perhaps become a bit fanatical with these (Crab Apple, Rock Water)? There may also be a lack of vitality (Hornbeam or Olive, depending on the depth of exhaustion).

Essences for Saturn Transiting Mercury

When under the hard transits of Saturn to our natal Mercury, our thinking and communication becomes more serious. Mercury symbolizes our thought and communication processes. Some change with these is now at hand. We feel the need of finding new ways of thinking and of expressing ourselves. Self-doubt about our ability to communicate (Larch) may arise, and some fear of successful communication (Mimulus). As we make these changes, we may feel misunderstood, withdraw into ourselves, and become silent (Agrimony). Depression may also set in, for our current mental state is colder and heavier (Gorse).

Essences for Saturn Transiting Venus

When under the hard transits of Saturn to our natal Venus, our values are re-examined. Venus symbolizes our concept of love and what we see as beautiful. During this period we are given the opportunity to see what is missing in our love life. This is not always easy, and we may discover that things are not going well. Feelings of depression may come up as we realize we are not getting the love we desire (Gorse), or we fear that our relationship is dissolving (Mimulus). Anger and resentment may now surface towards our partner (Willow), and we become critical and intolerant with him or her (Beech). Or we may totally repress our feelings to avoid the possibility of confrontation (Agrimony). Our self-confidence may also be at a low (Larch).

Essences for Saturn Transiting Mars

When under the hard transits of Saturn to our natal Mars, we become conscious of the way we use our energy. Mars symbolizes the way we take action. With Saturn's transit, we may find our actions held in limbo as we are taught the right use of action. We may feel afraid, or unable to accomplish something, during this period (Mimulus). Discouragement may set in, for we are beset by many setbacks and delays (Gentian). This is a time in which we may feel frustrated and stuck (Impatiens) and resent those whom we feel are holding us back (Willow). Struggle on one front or another will certainly take place, testing the limits of our endurance (Oak).

URANUS TRANSITS

Uranus symbolizes liberation and freedom. When Uranus comes a knockin', we are released from our old and rigid patterns in the way we have been living our lives. Change is the hallmark of this transit, although it may be quite sudden and unexpected, like a bolt of lightning out of the blue. This is a period when new insights and ways of handling old problems come to us. Issues of our uniqueness and individuality are brought to light with Uranus.

Essences for Uranus Transiting the Sun

When under the hard transits by Uranus to our natal Sun, we need plans A, B, and C! Nothing ever seems to go as planned, which may cause some initial discouragement (Gentian). Our very direction in life, or our identity, may be surprisingly changed, as we find dissatisfaction in what we have been doing (Wild Oat). We need to take care, however, that we don't "throw out the baby with the bath water" under this transit, as the energies unleashed are impulsive (Cherry Plum) and we feel quite detached (Water Violet). However, this is a time when we need to break from the past on some level, and bring changes into our lives (Walnut).

Essences for Uranus Transiting the Moon

When under the hard transits by Uranus to our natal Moon, our emotional nature is changed as we learn new ways of self-expression. Our emotional reactions may surprise us or others during this period. We find emotional reactions more difficult to control (Cherry Plum). We are easily irritated, or perhaps overly enthused (Impatiens, and possibly Vervain), and we are easily upset for no apparent reason (Mustard). Our emotional responses are quite unpredictable now, swinging one way and then the other (Scleranthus). Emotional detachment is also common (Water Violet).

Essences for Uranus Transiting Mercury

When under the hard transits by Uranus to our natal Mercury, changes in any rigid thinking and communication are in order. We may experience some mental stress or tension during this period, as our mind is working overtime (White Chestnut). Our mental stability may be questionable, due to the changes taking place (Scleranthus). Our minds are charged up as our mental processes are quickened, racing like a train out of control, and we may find miscommunication taking place with others (Impatiens, and Cherry Plum if we feel out of control). As a result, there may be a tendency to detach from others who don't understand us (Water Violet). Our minds are definitely wired and keyed up during this period (Vervain).

Essences for Uranus Transiting Venus

When under the hard transits by Uranus to our natal Venus, our ideas of love are changed, as well as what we value. Caution is advised in our impulsivity with new relationships: we are at risk of leaving an old one prematurely (Cherry Plum), as feelings of aloofness towards the current partner often take place (Water Violet). If we do leave, we may find that we've thrown the baby out with the bath water when this transit is over. Impatience with a present relationship is not uncommon (Impatiens); neither is intolerance (Beech). It is important, however, to re-examine what we have before rushing off in our overeagerness for the excitement of a new love (Vervain).

Essences for Uranus Transiting Mars

When under the hard transits by Uranus to our natal Mars, the way we take action is changed. Our behavior becomes unpredictable and erratic during this period, and we may take action before thinking (Cherry Plum), due in part to a sense of detachment from what we are doing (Water Violet). Our energy level is intensified as never before. We are impatient and hyper, with a build-up of physical tension that calls for release (Impatiens, Vervain).

NEPTUNE TRANSITS

Neptune symbolizes fantasy and delusion as well as inspiration.

During Neptune transits, all that is no longer needed is being dissolved. We also may feel ungrounded and a bit out of touch with reality during this time. Our energy level is also affected, and we are unable to accomplish as much as usual. Often, we feel a loss of hope and faith as we experience the dissolution of people and things that no longer serve us. Depression and a sense of isolation are common. Neptune transits are very subtle and nebulous. We are often unaware of what has been dissolved until the transit is over. During this time, we examine what is real, and what is illusory, in our lives. We are required to become more conscious.

Essences for Neptune Transiting the Sun

When under the hard transits by Neptune to our natal Sun, our very identity is slowly eroded. We sense that perhaps we have not been on course with our life, after all. We face confusion about who we are and what our purpose is (Wild Oat). We feel ungrounded, spacey, (Clematis) and bone tired (Olive), with our ability to focus and concentrate gone (White Chestnut). Fear may surface as our sense of clarity dissolves (Mimulus, and Aspen for anxiety) and we may feel hopelessness and loss (Gorse, Star). Panic may overcome us in the nebulousness we feel (Rock Rose). The temptation of self-medication with alcohol or drugs needs to be monitored (Cherry Plum).

Essences for Neptune Transiting the Moon

When under the hard transits by Neptune to our natal Moon, we feel emotionally vulnerable. Emotional loss and grief are highly possible under this transit (Star). Feelings of exhaustion are also common (Olive). A shift is taking place in our feeling nature. We are faced with what we have deluded ourselves about in the past, which may cause depression (Gorse) as well as self-blame and guilt (Pine). Feelings of lethargy and listlessness may result

(Wild Rose). Our world does not feel safe, and we may suffer from feelings of panic in the midst of our confusion (Rock Rose).

Essences for Neptune Transiting Mercury

When under the hard aspects by Neptune to our natal Mercury, we may fear that we are losing our minds (Cherry Plum), as Neptune brings its nebulousness to our thinking. We don't remember, from one minute to the next, where we have placed something. Our focus and concentration have also vanished (Clematis, White Chestnut). We may become impatient and irritable with our forgetfulness (Impatiens). Strange dreams and feelings of insecurity may bring on apprehension, anxiety, and panic (Aspen, Rock Rose).

Essences for Neptune Transiting Venus

When under the hard aspects by Neptune to our natal Venus, the rose-colored glasses will be removed. Illusions of love go with this transit, bringing feelings of loss (Star). We may fall in love with someone who is not right for us (usually a weak and needy individual whom we feel we can save) and realize our mistake too late (Cherry Plum, Chestnut Bud). We are not at our most discerning and are easily taken advantage of (Centaury); our common sense is nowhere to be found (Clematis). Under Neptune's influence we are searching for perfection. What we find is usually an illusion.

Essences for Neptune Transiting Mars

When under the hard aspects by Neptune to our natal Mars, the way we take action is affected. At times we may not know what we are doing (Clematis). There is a subtle draining of our energy level (Olive). Our sexual energies may be diverted, ranging from impotence to promiscuity. In either case, we are out of control (Cherry Plum). If we can't have good sex, depression may set in

(Gorse) as well as frustration, tension (Impatiens), and loss of self-esteem (Larch).

PLUTO TRANSITS

Pluto brings us the opportunity of transformation and regeneration, and symbolizes the death and rebirth process. This process is graphically illustrated by the mythic Phoenix, a bird that is consumed by fire, only to be resurrected from its own ashes. With Pluto we are forced to let go of people and situations that prevent our growth. Pluto's energy is evolutionary. We may not like it, but we have no choice in the matter.

Essences for Pluto Transiting the Sun

When under the hard transits by Pluto to our natal Sun, a new sense of identity is reborn. Our old identities go through a transformation process. For some of us, this is the dark night of the soul, and we feel the limits of our endurance have been reached (Sweet Chestnut). Our rigid patterns are broken, and relationships may end. This is often a painful process, with deep feelings of loss and grief (Star). We may try desperately to hold on, possessive and manipulative, jockeying for control in any way we know (Chicory). We struggle to no avail. The emotional devastation saps our strength (Olive) as we endure this struggle (Oak). Feelings of terror and panic may wash over us (Rock Rose). We feel vividly that we are going through a figurative death. We fear loss of security and feel foreboding, for we are powerless (Mimulus and Aspen) during this major upheaval towards personal transformation. As we experience necessary loss, we may find ourselves clinging to the past (Honeysuckle). Resentment or hatred towards those we think are responsible for our agony may consume us (Willow and Holly), inclining us to acts of revenge. We may turn this inward and be a danger to ourselves (Cherry Plum). This transit is most challenging to endure. Yet the Phoenix will rise and we will know the ordeal has been worthwhile.

Essences for Pluto Transiting the Moon

When under the hard transits by Pluto to our natal Moon, we experience an uprooting of our emotional nature. Old feelings and emotional issues of the past (and of childhood) now come up to be purged, released, and finally healed. We may feel out of control in our emotional reactions (Cherry Plum), endeavor to repress and deny our feelings (Agrimony), or become more emotionally demanding (Chicory). Our feelings are indeed intense, almost obsessional, during this period, and emotional tension is common (Impatiens). We are in a process of redefining our emotional nature by being plunged into its depths. This can bring up fear and apprehension (Mimulus, Aspen) as we come face to face with our primal urges, as well as our demons. Or, perhaps we may touch an inner rage that has been festering deep within us (Holly). Depression may also be a part of this experience as we uncover old emotional wounds (Gorse, Sweet Chestnut, Star) that must now be released and healed.

Essences for Pluto Transiting Mercury

When under the hard transits by Pluto to our natal Mercury, our thinking and communication processes transform. They may seem off balance (Scleranthus) while they are changing. Mental uncertainty, and insecurity in our thinking and communication, may throw us off center (Cerato, Mimulus). There may be stress, or panic, over this feeling of mental instability (Rock Rose), and a sense of losing our mind (Cherry Plum). Obsessive thinking may become a problem (White Chestnut). To defend our feelings of loss of mental control, we may become more controlling towards others (Chicory, Holly, Vervain, Vine).

Essences for Pluto Transiting Venus

When under the hard transits by Pluto to our natal Venus, ideas of what love is, as well as all that is appreciated and desired, are being transformed. We find our desire nature intensified, and feel a need to control and manipulate others to get what we want (Chicory). We may find ourselves out of control as well, with obsessive-compulsive behavior highly likely (Cherry Plum) as we strive to attain what we desire. Feelings of hope-lessness and loss may arise when we find our love object is unresponsive and may even leave us (Gorse, Star). With this transit we learn that we never can force another to love us. We may also attract a partner who is controlling toward us; out of our deep desire for love, we may allow ourselves to be manip-ulated and controlled (Centaury). Either way our concept of love is transformed into something higher.

Essences for Pluto Transiting Mars

When under the hard transits by Pluto to our natal Mars, an obsession for control in our actions now manifests, and we are vulnerable to taking excessive risks (Cherry Plum). As with all Pluto transits, intensity is keenly felt; with Mars involved, any repressed anger will now be unleashed into consciousness to be freed and healed. Some may respond by denying their feelings (Agrimony), and others by inappropriate expression (Willow, Holly, Cherry Plum). Our energy drive is also increased and there is a danger of overworking ourselves (Oak). If we have mismanaged our use of energy, this transit will teach us about right use of action.

I intend astrological information to provide you with another avenue of determining the flower essences that are appropriate for you. I trust you find this information advances your personal growth.

I leave you with some of Dr. Bach's thoughts on astrology and his flower essences. In an article from the September 1955 issue of *Astrology and Healing*, a Bach Flower Remedy newsletter, Dr. Bach tells us that the significance of the Remedies may be useful to those interested in the astrological side of healing. The planets symbolize the main battle for which we incarnated. They show the challenges we are to overcome. Dr. Bach assures us that the Divinity within each of us is stronger than the influences of any planet. The position of the planets in our charts, however, can show us our life's work and the reason for our birth. If we have challenging aspects, these are only indications that we are strong enough to be victorious. And so, the more difficult our chart may be, the greater will be our honor in overcoming these adversities. Dr. Bach goes on to say that the signs of the zodiac denote the personality we have chosen, the negative parts of our character that we must guard against, and the positive qualities that, when properly used, help us to gain the victory.

The birth chart of Dr. Bach is included in the Appendix. I felt this would interest readers who are astrologers. The date and place of Dr. Bach's birth are in Nora Weeks' book, *The Medical Discoveries of Edward Bach, Physician*. His time of birth was not mentioned in any of the literature I researched; I took the liberty of choosing the time that produced a natal chart that seemed to fit him and his life. I found it interesting to note that Dr. Bach's natal Moon was in the sign of Leo. He truly was an inspiring teacher.

In our next chapter we now turn to material on the chakra system, with the utilization of flower essences in facilitating chakra alignment and balance in our ongoing quest for wholeness.

8.

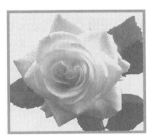

Supporting the Chakras

We need but close our eyes and feel the energy of
the…chakras, as the origin of our own power—as the
energy that fuels our biology. Ironically, once we realize
the stuff of which we are made, we have no choice but to
live a spiritual life.

—*Caroline Myss,* Anatomy of the Spirit

We can no longer ignore the supposition that the physical body
is but one in a series of interacting multidimensional subtle
energy systems. For too long, modern medicine has ignored this
possibility. Shortsightedly, physicians have only recognized and
treated the body and its symptoms. New evidence is mounting
that we are, indeed, comprised of networks of complex energy
fields that interface with our physical/cellular systems. The
body's subtle energy systems are now the subject of scientific
studies that have recognized the chakras and confirmed the
validity of ancient teachings regarding these subtle fields.

Our physical body is made up of sub-systems that support its
functioning—the circulatory system, nervous system, digestive
system, and the organs, tissues, cells, and so on, comprising

these. Our subtle fields have energy centers that support their functioning. These energy centers have come to be known as chakras, and are actually the link between body, mind, and spirit—between consciousness and the human form. For ages, adepts, seers, and intuitives have been aware of the chakra system. Many of them have the ability to see clairvoyantly these awesome spinning wheels of light emanating from within us.

The word "chakra" is Sanskrit, and literally means wheel. The chakras are described as spinning focal points of energy present in subtle matter. There are seven main chakras that function to receive, project, and transmit energy. They affect both the physical and subtle energy levels of the body. On the physical level, the chakras have been directly linked to the endocrine glands. They are located in the same areas, affecting these glands on subtle levels.

There is a strong correlation between the functioning of the chakras and our physical well-being, as each of the seven chakras reflects an aspect of consciousness essential to our lives. In most individuals, the chakras do not yet function at their optimum level. The three lower chakras—the Root, Navel, and Solar Plexus—are strongly connected to the personality, and the need to mature and become spiritualized. Yet, they are vital to our wholeness, and our life force must flow through these lower chakras to approach the higher ones. It is only when all the chakras are energized that a state of integration and wholeness between the personality and soul can be reached, culminating in humankind's ultimate goal of self-realization.

According to Anodea Judith, in *Wheels of Life*, a brilliant work on the chakras that I urge you to read, "From instinctual behavior to consciously planned strategies, from emotions to artistic creation, the chakras are the master programs that govern our life, loves, learning, and illumination. Like a rainbow bridge, they form the connecting channel between mind and body, spirit and matter, past and future, Heaven and Earth."

Each chakra is positioned behind an endocrine gland, beginning at the base of the spine where the First Chakra (Root Chakra) is found, interfacing with the adrenals. They continue vertically up through the body, culminating at the top of the head where the Seventh Chakra (Crown Chakra) is situated, interfacing with the pituitary. This is symbolic of our individual evolutionary process, moving through seven definite stages as we gain mastery over our lower self (our animal nature), and our higher self (spiritual nature) becomes fully integrated.

If we get stuck at any one stage, not addressing the need for growth called for in a particular chakra, its energy will eventually manifest in illness. This is usually located in and around the chakra area that has become blocked. Heart disease is a clear illustration of this process. When we think of love, the symbol of the heart most often comes to mind as an expression of this state. Some issue surrounding love is often directly related to heart problems. With heart disease, the corresponding Heart Chakra (interfacing with the thymus gland) is not functioning optimally, due to the individual's inability to love others or to love self. Perhaps someone is unable to forgive others or to forgive self. Other unresolved emotional issues can bring imbalance to the Heart Chakra. Should emotional disharmony continue, the onset of disease is certain.

The following is a brief delineation of the seven major chakras, indicating location, correlating endocrine gland, and the aspect of consciousness that relates to each. (See Figure 4 on the following page.)

THE SEVEN MAJOR CHAKRAS
Figure 4

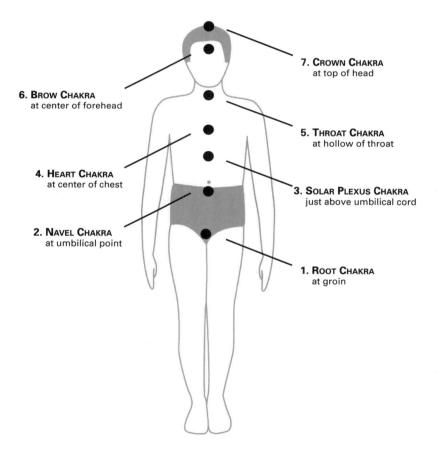

7. **CROWN CHAKRA**
at top of head

6. **BROW CHAKRA**
at center of forehead

5. **THROAT CHAKRA**
at hollow of throat

4. **HEART CHAKRA**
at center of chest

3. **SOLAR PLEXUS CHAKRA**
just above umbilical cord

2. **NAVEL CHAKRA**
at umbilical point

1. **ROOT CHAKRA**
at groin

THE SEVEN MAJOR CHAKRAS

Chakra	Location	Endocrine Gland	Consciousness
1st	Base of Spine	Adrenals	Survival
2nd	Just Below Navel (Female & Male Reproductive Organs)	Gonads	Desire
3rd	Solar Plexus	Pancreas	Personal Power
4th	Heart	Thymus	Love
5th	Throat	Thyroid	Communication/ Creativity
6th	Forehead	Pineal	Intuition
7th	Top of Head	Pituitary	Oneness

In the interest of wholeness and total health, it is important to consider the interconnection between the chakras and their potential effects upon the physical body. If an imbalance should develop in any chakra, there is a direct effect upon not only the endocrine gland associated with that chakra, but with the organ systems governed by that particular gland. This will create a potential for the manifestation of disease in that area. The previous example of heart disease aptly described this process.

As we saw in this example, chakra imbalances show up predominantly as deep-seated emotional issues, negative beliefs and attitudes, or personality flaws. Let us be aware of the importance of addressing and healing these before the advent of illness. Should any of these be left unchecked, the precipitation of a physical condition is assured. The perception that all illness begins above the material, before it filters down into the physical body, is key in our understanding and prevention of disease.

Let us now explore the chakras' life lessons (or functions), possible imbalances (emotional and mental issues), and associated physical malfunctions that may develop around these evolutionary patterns of growth.

The Functions (Life Lessons) and Issues of the Seven Chakras

1: Root Chakra

Muladhara is the Sanskrit name for the First Chakra. The color associated with this chakra is red, and it is positioned at the base of the spine. The vital life force (prana) is stored in this chakra. This energy flows upward to the Crown Chakra (Seventh Chakra), stimulating all the cells in every part of the body. The First Chakra functions to connect and ground us to the earth, so we are present in the body. It is concerned with basic security, survival, and existence.

Issues that surface here include family disengagement vs. group safety; ability to provide for and support oneself in the world; ability to protect and stand up for oneself; being connected to the earth, grounded, in order to function in the material. Possible physical malfunctions associated with the Root Chakra are obesity, anorexia, hemorrhoids, constipation, chronic fatigue, problems with the lower extremities, bones, large intestines.

2: Navel Chakra

Svadhisthana is the Sanskrit name for the Second Chakra. The color associated with this chakra is orange, and it is positioned just below the navel. The main function of the Navel Chakra is desire. This is the seat of our emotions, with our feelings running rampant until we mature and learn to control them.

Issues that surface here include sexuality and sexual identity; money; emotional nurturance; power and control in relationships; socialization; commitment; manipulation; blame and guilt; procreation. Possible physical malfunctions associated with the Navel Chakra are impotence, frigidity, infertility, prostate, testicular, ovarian, or uterine difficulties, bladder and kidney problems.

3: Solar Plexus Chakra

Manipura is the Sanskrit name for the Third Chakra. The color associated with this chakra is yellow, and it is positioned in the solar plexus. The main function of the Solar Plexus Chakra is personal power. It is the seat of our self-confidence. Its energy allows us to accomplish and achieve.

Issues that surface here include trust in others; intimidation and domination (from or over others); power and control; self-esteem; decision making; sensitivity to criticism; influence of others; personal honor. Possible physical malfunctions associated with the Solar Plexus Chakra are ulcers, diabetes, hypoglycemia, digestive, pancreatic, and adrenal problems.

4: Heart Chakra

Anahata is the Sanskrit name for the Fourth Chakra. The color associated with this Chakra is green, and it is positioned in the chest. This is the center of unconditional love; the main function of the Heart Chakra is compassion and caring—for self as well as others. This is considered the Master Chakra, and when it is fully functioning the power of love becomes the motivating force in our lives. The Heart Chakra is the opening of higher consciousness and the higher self, where wisdom and love merge.

Issues that surface here include love and hatred; resentment and bitterness; grief and anger; self-centeredness; loneliness and isolation; forgiveness and compassion; trust. Possible physical malfunctions associated with the Heart Chakra are high blood pressure, asthma, lung, and heart problems.

5: Throat Chakra

Visshudha is the Sanskrit name for the Fifth Chakra. The color associated with this chakra is light blue, and it is positioned in the throat. The main function of the Throat Chakra is communication and the expression of creativity.

Issues that surface here include personal expression and creativity; speaking one's truth; choice and strength of will; following one's dream; addiction; judgment and criticism of others; capacity to make decisions. Possible physical malfunctions associated with the Throat Chakra are hypo- and hyperthyroidism, ear, throat, and mouth problems, stuttering, neck, and upper shoulder pain.

6: Brow Chakra

Ajna is the Sanskrit name for the Sixth Chakra. The color associated with this chakra is indigo, and it is positioned between the eyes. The main function of the Brow Chakra is clear vision and intuition. In many individuals, this chakra lies dormant. It is usually used in our judgment of self and of others until it is awakened. With the spiritualization of this chakra, both hemispheres of the brain are integrated, creating balance between our female and male energies.

Issues that surface here include self-evaluation; truth; intellectual abilities; personal competence; openness to ideas of others; ability to learn from mistakes; use of the imagination; perception. Possible physical malfunctions associated with the Brow Chakra are cataracts, glaucoma, blindness, general problems with vision, headaches, nightmares.

7: Crown Chakra

Sahasrara is the Sanskrit name for the Seventh Chakra. The color associated with this chakra is violet, and it is positioned at the top of the head. The main function of the Crown Chakra is that of unity and the oneness of all life—that we are all one. This chakra is also dormant in most individuals. Once it is opened we sense our purpose, and recognize that, indeed, we are a divine child of God. And we are here to share our light, love, and wisdom with our younger (in evolution) brothers and sisters. The soul's role as co-creator is now felt.

Issues that surface here include one's values, ethics, humanitarianism; selflessness; ability to see the larger picture and trust life; faith and inspiration; spirituality and devotion. Possible physical malfunctions associated with the Crown Chakra are depression, alienation, confusion, and problems related to the brain.

We can clearly see that there is an impressive correlation between the emotional and mental issues associated with the chakras and the negative states of mind that the Bach Flower Essences treat. Flower essences can be used to reinstate harmony and balance to our chakra system and prevent disease. It is obvious that flower essences have far-reaching effects on many levels.

With our grasp of the issues concerning each of the chakras, let us next address the Bach Flowers that correspond to these so we may facilitate our healing process on a deeper level, furthering personal growth.

RESTORING CHAKRA BALANCE WITH THE BACH FLOWERS

NOTE: The emotional issues for each of the chakras are offered again as we explore the flower essences that assist in healing these.

The First Chakra

The Root Chakra's primary function is survival. Issues here often have their inception in early childhood, when our dependency needs are not adequately met. We learn to see the world as an unsafe place. The only world we knew as an infant, our immediate family, did not provide for us. We may grow up with deep-seated feelings of fear, mistrust, and resentment, or we may be unable to set boundaries and stand up for ourselves. We may feel incapable of taking care of ourselves, being unable to break away from the dysfunctional family patterns that have ingrained themselves within us. Being in touch with and grounded in the physical, as well as accepting the body and caring for its needs, are also First Chakra functions.

The flower essences Mimulus (for fear), Holly (for mistrust), Willow (for resentment), Centaury (for not standing up for oneself), Larch (for low self-esteem), and Walnut (to protect against outside influences) strongly relate to First Chakra issues. Agrimony (to release inner torment that has been repressed) may also be considered, as well as Honeysuckle (to release the past), if haunting childhood memories are a concern. Star of Bethlehem should also be regarded for any childhood abuse that took place. Also consider Clematis (not being in the present moment as well as not grounded in the body) and Honeysuckle (for living in the past and being out of touch with present needs). Crab Apple is indicated for deep-seated issues of shame, physical self-disgust, and in some instances, is indicated for eating disorders such as anorexia and bulimia, which may culminate in starvation and possible death.

Obesity is also connected to the First Chakra. Issues that may lead to obesity are poor self-esteem (Larch), self-condemnation (Crab Apple), fear of intimacy and self-protection (Mimulus), self-blame, and guilt (Pine). These essences may be helpful in treating the core issues. Other flower essences to consider in dealing with the emotional effects of obesity are Agrimony (for self-medicating with food, putting on a brave front, as well as denial of feelings), Wild Rose (for apathy and resignation with this condition), Willow (for resentment towards others' judgment), or Gorse (for hopelessness). Also consider Cherry Plum (for loss of control with eating), Chestnut Bud (to break the habit pattern of this self-destructive behavior), or Gentian (for despair with setbacks and delays with dieting).

The Second Chakra

The Navel Chakra's primary function is desire (emotions), sexuality, and nurturance. Relationships and relating to others (socialization), blame and guilt, money and sex, power and control (manipulation), procreation, and ethics and honor in relationships are the issues that are associated with the Second Chakra.

The flower essences that correlate to these issues are Agrimony (for the inability to confront others); Beech (for intolerance); Centaury (for lack of boundaries and allowing others to be abusive); Chestnut Bud (for failure to learn from past mistakes); Cherry Plum (addressing lust, sexual obsession, and other misuse of sexual energy); Chicory (for possessiveness, selfishness, and manipulation); Crab Apple (for issues of shame); Holly (for jealousy and mistrust); Heather (for self-involvement); Impatiens (for cruelty); Mimulus (for fear of intimacy); Pine (for self-blame and guilt); Vervain (for always needing to be right); Vine (for domination and inflexibility); Water Violet (for pride and detachment); and Willow (for bitterness).

The Third Chakra

The Solar Plexus Chakra's primary function is personal power. Issues here surround trust, fear, and intimidation (as well as intimidating others), power and control, greed, envy, self-worth, confidence in decision making, judgment, and criticism.

The flower essences that correlate to Third Chakra issues are Agrimony (for the inability to confront others); Beech (for being critical, judgmental); Centaury (for allowing oneself to be taken advantage of); Cerato (for doubting one's own judgment); Cherry Plum (addressing aggressiveness, intimidation); Chicory (for manipulation); Gentian (for lack of faith with setbacks and delays); Holly (for suspicion, revenge, jealousy, envy); Larch (for low self-esteem, self-confidence, self-respect); Mimulus (addressing fear of intimidation); Oak (for pushing oneself too hard); Vervain (always having to be right and needing to win); Vine (being dictatorial, greed for power and control); Wild Rose (for lack of motivation); Walnut (being easily influenced by others).

The Fourth Chakra

The Heart Chakra's primary function is love and compassion—for self as well as others. Issues here surround love and hatred, resentment and bitterness, loneliness and isolation, commitment, grief and anger, forgiveness and compassion, self-centeredness, selfishness, possessiveness, hope and trust, and self-acceptance.

The flower essences that correlate to Fourth Chakra issues are Beech (for intolerance, instilling compassion); Centaury (unable to consider personal needs, giving self away, co-dependent); Chicory (for selfish love); Crab Apple (for self-disgust, non-acceptance of the physical body); Gentian (for lack of faith); Heather (for self-centeredness); Holly (for hatred, jealousy, envy, mistrust, lack of compassion, heart has been closed); Impatiens (for cruelty); Larch (for feelings of inferiority); Mimulus (addressing fear of commitment, of rejection); Pine (addressing self-perfection, guilt); Red Chestnut (for overconcern); Rock Water (addressing self-denial, martyrdom); Star of Bethlehem (for grief); Vervain (for egocentricity); Vine (being controlling); Water Violet (for pride and detachment); Willow (for bitterness and resentment).

The Fifth Chakra

The Throat Chakra's primary function is communication and creativity. Issues here surround choice and strength of will, personal expression, following one's dreams, creativity, addiction, judgment and criticism, faith, capacity to make decisions, and finding one's voice.

The flower essences that correlate to Fifth Chakra issues are Agrimony (releasing repressed issues, inability to speak up and confront others); Beech (to release judgment and criticism towards others); Centaury (being weak-willed); Cerato (to instill self-confidence in decision making); Agrimony, Cherry Plum, Chestnut Bud, and Walnut (for addictions: Agrimony to release repression and denial of feelings that lead to self-medication, Cherry Plum for loss of control, Chestnut Bud for negative repetitive behavior patterns, and Walnut as the "link breaker" for assisting with transition); Clematis (being ungrounded and unable to bring creativity into practicality); Gentian (to instill faith with setbacks and delays); Impatiens (for lack of patience); Larch (to instill self-confidence in personal creativity); Mimulus (for fear in self-expression and of being judged); Pine (for demanding too much of self—only perfection); Rock Water (for being too hard on self, rigid); Walnut (to be able to follow one's dream and not be influenced by others); White Chestnut (to still the restless mind and bring focus and concentration to one's creative process); Wild Oat (when purpose in life is uncertain); and Wild Rose (for apathy and resignation).

The Sixth Chakra

The Brow Chakra's primary function is perception and intuition. Issues here surround self-evaluation, truth, intellectual ability, feelings of personal competence , openness to the ideas of others, ability to learn from experience, use of the imagination, and perception.

The flower essences that correlate to Sixth Chakra issues are Beech (to release judgment and criticism towards others); Cerato (for trusting one's own decisions and inner wisdom); Clematis (for being lost in a world of fantasy, carried away with imaginings, delusions, as well as for needing to ground one's intuition and make it practical); Chestnut Bud (to be able to learn from past mistakes); Crab Apple (for feelings of physical imperfection); Larch (for feelings of inadequacy, poor self-image); Pine (for self-blame); Scleranthus (to bring confidence in making choices); Vervain and Vine (for being opinionated and inflexible, domineering and rigid, instilling flexibility and openness to the ideas of others); Walnut (to follow one's inner truth and ideals, to be unaffected by others' opinions); White Chestnut (to quiet the mind and be in touch with one's intuition); Willow (to be able to see personal responsibility for one's own life and release resentment towards others).

The Seventh Chakra

The Crown Chakra's primary function is unity and oneness with all life. Issues here encompass one's values, ethics, humanitarianism, selflessness, the ability to see the larger picture and trust life, to have faith and inspiration, spirituality and devotion.

The flower essences that correlate to Seventh Chakra issues are Aspen (for feelings of foreboding and apprehension); Beech (for judging others); Chicory (for selfishness and possessiveness); Gentian (for instilling faith and trust in the grand scheme of life when things don't go as planned); Gorse (instilling hope when all hope is gone); Heather (turning self-concern to empathy for others); Holly (for mistrust); Honeysuckle (for releasing the past and moving forward); Mimulus (to instill courage in the face of doubt and fear); Sweet Chestnut (for the dark night of the soul, bringing back the light); Vine and Vervain (being pushy and controlling, being egocentric and not considering others' needs); Water Violet (for the sense of detachment and noninvolvement, to assist in relating to others and sharing one's gifts); Walnut (to protect against the influence of others, being undeterred from following one's own inspiration and path in life).

We have completed our review of the chakra system, and of the flower essences that relate to the multifaceted issues involved with each of the seven chakras. We can see that many of the issues we face and need to grow through are not necessarily confined to a single chakra. As you have probably observed, several chakras share facets of this learning process on different levels. We are complex and unique individuals. It is almost impossible to synthesize, simply and easily, the intricacies that permeate our beings. We can only do our best to truly know ourselves, to uncover both our strengths and our weaknesses, and to be willing to continue with our process of self-discovery. At the very least, we now have a place to start. And with the flower essences, we have been given a gentle, simple, and safe approach to facilitate and promote our personal growth and emotional healing.

In our final chapter, we explore the practice of meditation. A commitment to a daily practice of meditation is one of the most important techniques that I know to increase and maintain your state of health to the highest degree. I share this information in the interest of providing you with as many ways as possible towards this end.

9.

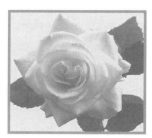

Meditation

Be still and know that I am God.

—Psalm 46:10

I felt strongly compelled to provide information on meditation before concluding this book. I would be remiss in not making you aware of the profound influence meditation has on the chakra system and how this practice facilitates chakra attunement and balance. Those of you who are seeking to advance your personal healing process and your spiritual growth will find wonderful support by incorporating the practice of meditation into your daily life.

The idea of relaxing and taking time to meditate goes against our training. We live in a left-brained world. We have been conditioned by our Western society to be active and productive. Time for contemplation is not honored. *Doing* is held in high esteem, and *being* is frowned upon. Many think that meditation is a nonproductive enterprise.

To our detriment, we rarely use the right brain, which is receptive and the seat of one's intuition and creativity. We are mostly a left-brained society that is ruled by logic. We are missing out on so much by assigning a less valuable role to our imagination and intuitive sensings. Part of our becoming whole is in learning to use both hemispheres of the brain equally, allowing both the analytical, logical half and the receptive, intuitive half to coexist in cooperation and harmony. To do this requires taking time each day to be still, to meditate—to just be. After all, we are human beings, not human doings.

The practice of meditation is one of the most effective methods for creating balance between the right and left sides of the brain. It is also a means of opening to, and supporting, our spirituality—where the still, small voice may be heard. In meditation, we are also initiating the process of attuning the chakras. In this harmonization, the chakras empower the connection between the personality and the soul. The stronger this link becomes, enhanced by the daily practice of meditation, the more the personality is in tune to the soul's purpose and life path. And it is precisely this balance and harmony that is necessary for optimum maintenance of our total health and well-being.

For this reason all the great masters and seers of the past ages have advocated the practice of meditation and have spoken of our seeking the silence. They knew that meditation is one of the surest ways of promoting health, as well as in finding peace and enlightenment. As mentioned in an earlier chapter, Dr. Bach himself was a proponent of meditation. In *Heal Thyself*, he wrote of the importance of uncovering our personality flaws as well as our hidden strengths. He counseled that the practice of meditation was the perfect method for discovering these. Taking the time to be still each day, we are given an avenue to knowing ourselves more intimately, and to receiving guidance from a higher source.

Meditation has transpersonal benefits, but taking at least fifteen minutes a day to tune out the turmoil of the world is of itself beneficial. Meditation assists us in relieving the anxiety, pressure, stress, and tension of our everyday life. By tuning out and turning within, we are returned to our natural state of inner peace, balance, and harmony.

There are many wonderful books available on meditation, and it is easily self-taught. To give you a sense of just how simple it is, and perhaps to inspire and motivate you before you have the opportunity to pick up a book, I will offer some basic guidelines for meditating. I trust that as you go along, you will develop your own techniques. Meditation styles can be as simple or intricate as you choose, and the only right way is your way. It is important to recognize that we are all unique individuals. What is right for one is not necessarily right for another. Allow yourself to experiment and to find the meditation technique that is appropriate for you.

Regarding our individuality and uniqueness, it is also important not to have any pre-set expectations as to what your meditation experience may be. It will be different for each of us. Please also be aware that the true purpose of meditation is not in seeing visions or hearing voices, although some may experience these. Many times, these are distractions from entering the silence, where the peace that passes all understanding is found, and what we are truly seeking. Please don't put pressure on yourself, if it seems that nothing is happening for you. Know that on very subtle levels a great deal is taking place, regardless of any lack of conscious awareness.

General guidelines now follow to initiate and facilitate your introductory meditation experience. You take it from here.

INSTRUCTION FOR MEDITATION

Find a comfortable and quiet location that will become your meditation space, somewhere you can go to be alone and undisturbed. Let others know that when you are meditating, you are not to be interrupted (unless, of course, a dire emergency should arise). If this is not possible, perhaps you can meditate when no one else is home, or late in the evening, or early in the morning while others are still asleep.

Initially, it is also helpful to establish a particular time each day, in order to set a new routine more easily. In this way you give your body and mind the firm message that this is now part of your daily regime. And they'll be more likely to cooperate and be less resistant.

Whenever we take on a new discipline, an exercise program or new diet for example, at first there may be a part of us that resists. Be aware that this is natural. As you probably know well, resistance to change is part of the human experience. Just move through any resistance if you find this happening to you. Your commitment is essential. It is only by holding to your discipline and taking it seriously that you will be able to finally achieve and experience success.

Once you've established the location and time for your meditation practice, and are wearing loose and comfortable clothing, you are ready to begin. Sit in a relaxed position, making sure that your spine is straight (for chakra alignment). Keep your legs uncrossed, feet touching the floor (unless you opt to sit in lotus position), and place your hands (palms up) on your lap. Close your eyes and allow yourself to move into a space of total relaxation as you let go of any remaining cares and concerns.

You may find listening to soft, gentle music helpful in creating an atmosphere more conducive to fully relaxing. Lighting a candle and/or use of incense is also supportive. Above all, a sense of reverence is of the utmost importance. Realize that you are creating a sacred space to commune with your Creator. You may find taking a moment or two in a simple prayer of gratitude to be quite helpful in setting the tone.

Once you relax into your space of calm and quiet, allow yourself to observe your body. Get a feel for any tension that may be present, and gently suggest to yourself that you are now letting it go. Begin at the top of your head and slowly move down your body, releasing any remaining tension you may find. Once you've created a state of relaxation, begin to follow your breathing. Your breath will now become the focal point throughout your meditation.

Concentrating on the breath assists in closing off all unwanted thoughts. In normal waking consciousness, the mind is forever jumping from one thought to another. Our heads are filled with constant chatter, whether we realize it or not. The purpose of meditation is to create a still and quiet mind. It is in this stillness that the door is opened to another level of reality, the very existence of which we are seldom aware of. If you find yourself thinking about something else, just bring your attention back to the breath once more—as many times as necessary.

Please be patient with yourself when you find your mind wandering. And it will, as this is common in the beginning. With practice and time, your distractions will fade, your focus will increase, and your meditation become deeper and richer. For added assistance in quieting the mind, consider the Bach Flower, *White Chestnut*. This flower essence is extremely helpful in supporting your concentration and focus. You may want to take a few drops before you begin.

Continue to observe your breath coming in and going out through your nose. Is it warm? Is it cool? Just be with your breath. Don't try to control the pace of your breathing. As you continue to follow the breath, you will find it slowing down and becoming more rhythmic on its own. Go with its natural flow.

You can then add, if you choose, a personal affirmation. The use of an affirmation can assist in sustaining the focus of your concentration. You do not need to say your affirmation aloud; simply repeat it silently to yourself as you breathe.

To illustrate, let us take one of my personal favorites, *"Be still and know that I am God."* On the in-breath repeat, "Be still and know." On the out-breath repeat, "that I am God." You may use any other affirmation you choose. It may be a single word, such as peace, love, or any other word or phrase that brings a sense of comfort to you. Please work with whatever is meaningful to you. Also know that you do not need to use an affirmation. It is simply another tool that facilitates a strong focus. Following the breath itself will be sufficient to bring about the altered state of consciousness you are seeking. And remember, please relax and just go with the flow.

Remain with your focused breathing for five to ten minutes in the beginning. You will find this length of time enough of a challenge to start with. Both the body and the mind will typically protest at first, until they get the idea you are really serious. You may feel fidgety, and your mind will think up the most amazing thoughts to distract your attention. When this happens, just gently, but firmly, re-focus your mind back to the breath and/or affirmation being used. Little by little, you will find the body and mind no longer resisting your practice. When you are ready, you may increase the length of time. Intuitively you will know how long is right for you.

As we take on a meditative discipline, most of us are not used to being quiet and still. We generally live a life filled with many responsibilities that require our constant attention and energy. It may feel a bit uncomfortable, at first, to shift your attention and allow yourself this luxury of just letting go for a short while. Yet, know it is more than a luxury. It is a vital part of self-care that you do deserve. And I guarantee that whatever you've left undone will still be waiting for you. But by taking this break from the stress and tension in your life, you will find new strength and clarity to support your endeavors.

When you feel you've spent five or ten minutes in silence, I highly recommend that you make use of the energy that has been evoked while in this state, and now offer prayers of healing to those you feel are in need. Simply visualize or sense a healing light surrounding and permeating the body of each individual you are praying for. Imagine their face in your mind's eye and see them relaxed and at peace. It is important not to specify the way in which any healing is to take place. As this is truly God's domain, our prayer is solely, *Thy Will Be Done*. Only God, and the soul of the individual you are praying for, know how this energy is best utilized. In this manner, you are facilitating another's healing process with your prayer in a way that is non-interfering. Be assured that the energy sent will be used as needed, and it will be right and perfect for that individual.

After completing your healing prayers for others, please take a few moments for your own healing as well. Again, with the use of visualization, sense the healing light now surrounding yourself. Allow this energy to fill your entire being. Stay with this for as long as feels comfortable. Once completed, slowly and gently bring yourself back to normal consciousness. Draw your awareness back to your body. Feel how solid it is as you become centered and grounded once more in the physical. Move your fingers and toes, take a deep breath, and open your eyes when ready. Give yourself a few moments before getting up, as you may experience some dizziness, which is perfectly normal.

What has just been described is one of numerous methods in meditation practice. I would like to offer another approach you may find helpful in asking for specific guidance. With this method, we meditate with *intention*. The major difference in this approach concerns our focus. Instead of focusing on the breath alone, we now bring in a specific question or problem that needs clarity, and hold this in our consciousness. As we offer our issue up, we trust that a solution is coming, and we are open to receiving the answer. Keep in mind that guidance may not always come during the meditation process itself. You may receive a vivid and pointed dream, or you may suddenly receive intuitive knowledge, in the middle of your busy schedule. I have received remarkable guidance while driving my car. I have learned to keep a pen and pad handy in order to jot this information down.

Meditating with intention may also be helpful when you don't know which flower essences you need, or are uncertain of which flower essences to select. Bring these questions into your meditation for assistance whenever you feel stuck. My higher guidance has stepped in many times while I was dreaming, vividly alerting me to a particular essence I had need of, but was not currently using. These experiences have been eye-openers—right on target. The use of intention while meditating may also help you determine your type flower essence—the flower essence(s) that reflects your core personality. This may not be clear initially. Simply request in your meditation that guidance be given to you regarding your type essence(s), and know the answer will soon appear in one form or another.

Keeping a dream journal is an excellent idea. Many times we are given fabulous guidance while dreaming. Yet, we either forget our dream upon awakening or simply ignore it, unaware of the rich source of guidance that a dream may hold. By capturing in your journal whatever bits and pieces of a dream you do remember, you are better able to tune in to whatever messages may be present. By keeping a dream journal, you are also alerting your higher Source that you are now paying attention to your dreams. As you continue to work with your dreams, recognizing them as an avenue for direction, your dreams will be easier to remember.

Going into a meditative state just after taking a particular essence may also be an exercise to consider. In this way, a deeper understanding of the state of balance a particular essence provides may be revealed to you. When I was training in the use and practice of Bach Flowers, we undertook this exercise as one way to sense the energies of the flower essences. Each day, for thirty-eight days, we agreed to only use a single essence, starting alphabetically with Agrimony and finishing with Willow. In the evening, as we took our last dose, we would spend several minutes or so in a meditative state, mindful of whatever energy we might feel. Essence by essence, we were able to experience the subtle and unique vibration in each of the flower essences separately. We also kept a journal to record what we experienced with each essence. This exercise was most profound, and I found it to increase my personal sensitivity to what the flower essences hold. This may be a helpful exercise for you as well. If you don't feel the need to go through all thirty-eight as I did, it certainly would be beneficial to practice this exercise with those essences you are currently using.

As we now come to the end of this chapter on meditation, I trust any previous mystery or concerns have been dispelled. Meditation is really a quite simple and almost effortless process that any of us can easily incorporate into our daily life. The process is short and simple, and it is so very worthwhile to make this small effort in the interest of greater well-being. I encourage, and even urge, you not to hesitate a moment longer in initiating your personal meditation practice. It will forever change your life. You will experience a more relaxed and centered state of being, and, with the shift taking place in consciousness, you will find your dreams becoming a rich source of guidance and your intuitive abilities expanding. Most significantly, you will find your connection to spirit growing deeper, stronger, and more accessible.

In regard to the importance of meditation for chakra alignment, I have created a profound guided meditation, *To Touch the Light*. This audio program was designed specifically to empower your seven energy centers. To order your personal copy to facilitate your ongoing chakra attunement, please see the Resource section.

In concluding this chapter, I leave you with familiar words that express my heartfelt sentiments to you all. In the immortal words of *Star Trek's* Mr. Spock, "May you live long and prosper…"

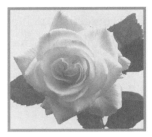

A Final Note

...Hence it may be truly said that to be at-variance (to the divine law) may bring sickness, disease, disruption, distress in a physical body...O that all would gain just that! and not feel, "Yes, I understand—but my desires and my body and my weaknesses and this or that—and I didn't do it" Who else did? This may be a hard statement for many, but you will eventually come to know it is true: No fault, no hurt comes to self save that thou hast created in thine consciousness, in thine inner self, the cause...

—Edgar Cayce, Reading 262-83

My purpose in writing this text has been threefold: to educate, to inspire, and to create change in my desire to empower you, dear reader, in relation to your health. For too many years we have given our power away to the health profession in regard to our personal healing. And in truth, our healing is personal—so much more personal than we ever imagined. The understanding and recognition that we are our own healers must finally be acknowledged. That the power lies within us is what I have desired to bring home to you. Realize that it is not enough to care for the physical body alone. To truly maintain our well-being, the care of the mind and spirit must also be addressed. And we can clearly see the importance of also maintaining our health on a daily basis, with preventative care on all levels—before the onset of disease. For, in our everyday life, how we attend to our physical, mental, emotional, and spiritual components impacts our health and the integrity of our total energetic system, literally for good or ill.

The time has come to know that we are so much more than we can see, that our physical bodies are only one in a multidimensional system of other bodies intertwined, no matter how subtle they may be. Preserving balance, mentally and emotionally, is key in promoting our well-being. Beyond this, we need to embrace our spirituality. Down through the ages we have been urged, not only by Dr. Bach, but by many other notable, wise, and inspired teachers, who have given us the very same message: Personality and soul alignment is necessary to maintaining our health and happiness in this life.

I trust that my purpose has been accomplished, and you have come to see yourself in a new light. I hope you now recognize, in defining who you are, that your physical body is just the tip of the iceberg. You are a spiritual being, primarily. The body and mind are miraculous instruments through which your soul may evolve on its journey to wholeness. Harmony between all three—body, mind, and spirit—is imperative in gaining and maintaining an optimum state of health. Truly, as the renowned twentieth century psychic, Edgar Cayce, teaches us, *"Spirit is the life, mind is the builder, and the physical is the result."* Let us be mindful that health ultimately does not depend upon medical practices. It depends on us, and our learning to live in a whole, harmonic, and loving way in every aspect of our lives. And as we do this, our bodies will respond with a constant rebalancing, healing, and regeneration of ourselves.

The challenge offered to you at this point is to be willing to take personal charge of your life as never before, to now address *more* than the physical body, in your personal quest for health and well-being. We must begin to heal dis-ease and distress at the level of *cause*. In order to work with vibrational healing methods, we must be ready to also move towards personal transformation. Know that this is a necessary first step before true physical and spiritual healing can manifest. The choice is yours…

In loving, healing light,
Rachelle

We must be steadfast in the determination to win, resolute in the will to gain the mountain summit; let us not give a moment's regret to the slips by the way. No great ascent was ever made without faults and falls, and they must be regarded as experiences which will help us to stumble less in the future. No thoughts of past errors must ever depress us; they are over and finished, and the knowledge thus gained will help to avoid a repetition of them. Steadily must we press forwards and onwards, never regretting and never looking back, for the past of even one hour ago is behind us, and the glorious future with its blazing light ever before us. All fear must be cast out; it should never exist in the human mind, and is only possible when we lose sight of our Divinity. It is foreign to us because as Sons of the Creator, Sparks of Divine Life, we are invincible, indestructible and unconquerable.

—*Edward Bach,* Heal Thyself

Bach Flower Keyword
Indications by Category

Flower Essence	Keyword Indications	Page
1. Fear		
Rock Rose	Panic, terror	33
Mimulus	Known fear	33
Cherry Plum	Fear of loss of control	34
Aspen	Unknown fear, foreboding	34
Red Chestnut	Fear, overconcern for loved ones	35
2. Uncertainty		
Cerato	Uncertainty in decision-making	36
Scleranthus	Indecision, vacillation	37
Gentian	Discouraged by setbacks, delays	37
Gorse	Hopelessness	39
Hornbeam	Lack of strength, low vitality	40
Wild Oat	Uncertain of path in life	41
3. Insufficient Interest in Present Circumstances		
Clematis	Dreamy, living in the future	41
Honeysuckle	Nostalgic, living in the past	42
Wild Rose	Apathy, resignation	42
Olive	Extreme exhaustion	43
White Chestnut	Restless mind, obsessive thoughts	44
Mustard	Depression from unknown origin	44
Chestnut Bud	Failure to learn from the past	44

Botanical Names of
the 38 Bach Flower Essences

Flower Essence	**Botanical Name**
Agrimony	*Agrimonia eupatoria*
Aspen	*Populus tremula*
Beech	*Fagus sylvatica*
Centaury	*Centaurium umbellatum*
Cerato	*Ceratostigma willmottiana*
Cherry Plum	*Prunus cerasifera*
Chestnut Bud	*Aesculus hippocastanum*
Chicory	*Cichorium intybus*
Clematis	*Clematis vitalba*
Crab Apple	*Malus sylvestris*
Elm	*Ulmus procera*
Gentian	*Gentiana amarella*
Gorse	*Ulex europoeus*
Heather	*Calluna vulgaris*
Holly	*Ilex aquifolium*
Honeysuckle	*Lonicera caprifolium*
Hornbeam	*Carpinus betulus*
Impatiens	*Impatiens glandulifera*
Larch	*Larix decidua*
Mimulus	*Mimulus guttatus*

Flower Essence	Botanical Name
Mustard	*Sinapis arvensis*
Oak	*Quercus robur*
Olive	*Olea europoea*
Pine	*Pinus sylvestris*
Red Chestnut	*Aesculus carnea*
Rock Rose	*Helianthemum nummularium*
Rock Water	*Aqua petra**
Scleranthus	*Scleranthus annuus*
Star of Bethlehem	*Ornithogalum umbetelatum*
Sweet Chestnut	*Castanea sativa*
Vervain	*Verbena officinalis*
Vine	*Vitis vinifera*
Walnut	*Juglans regia*
Water Violet	*Hottonia palustris*
White Chestnut	*Aesculus hippocastanum*
Wild Oat	*Bromus ramosus*
Wild Rose	*Rosa canina*
Willow	*Salix vitellina*

*Rock Water is the only Bach Essence that is not made from flowering trees or plants. It comes from healing waters near Dr. Bach's home.

Virtues of
the 38 Bach Flower Essences

Flower Essence	Virtue
Agrimony	Joyfulness
Aspen	Fearlessness
Beech	Tolerance
Centaury	Self-determination
Cerato	Inner Certainty
Cherry Plum	Composure
Chestnut Bud	Capacity for Learning
Chicory	Selfless Love
Clematis	Creative Idealism
Crab Apple	Purity
Elm	Right Responsibility
Gentian	Faith
Gorse	Hope
Heather	Empathy
Holly	Unconditional Love
Honeysuckle	Capacity for Change
Hornbeam	Inner Vitality
Impatiens	Patience
Larch	Self-confidence

Flower Essence	**Virtue**
Mimulus	Courage
Mustard	Cheerfulness
Oak	Endurance
Olive	Regeneration
Pine	Forgiveness
Red Chestnut	Solicitude
Rock Rose	Steadfastness
Rock Water	Adaptability
Scleranthus	Balance
Star of Bethlehem	Restoration
Sweet Chestnut	Release
Vervain	Restraint
Vine	Right Use of Authority
Walnut	Unaffectedness
Water Violet	Humility
White Chestnut	Tranquility
Wild Oat	Purposefulness
Wild Rose	Inner Motivation
Willow	Personal Responsibility

Birth Chart of
Dr. Edward Bach

*Note—The exact hour of Dr. Bach's birth, on September 24, 1886, is unknown. Based on my intuition that he was a Virgo Rising, I have selected 5:45 am as the time of birth.

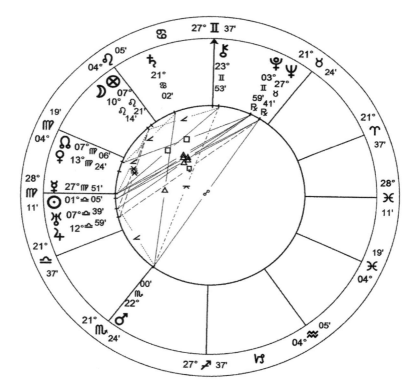

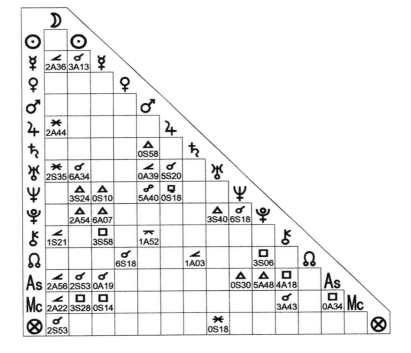

Bach Flower "Type" Essences for Natal Moon Signs

Natal Moon Sign	Corresponding "Type" Flower Essence
Aries	Impatiens
Taurus	Gentian
Gemini	Cerato
Cancer	Clematis
Leo	Vervain
Virgo	Centaury
Libra	Scleranthus
Scorpio	Chicory
Sagittarius	Agrimony
Capricorn	Mimulus
Aquarius	Water Violet
Pisces	Rock Rose

Resources for Further Study

BOOKS

Bach Flower Essences

Bach, Dr. Edward & Wheeler, Dr. F.J. *The Bach Flower Remedies.* New Canaan, CT: Keats Publishing Co., 1979.

Bernard, Julian (Editor). *Collected Writings of Edward Bach.* Worcester, England: Ebenezer Baylis, 1987.

Hasnas, Rachelle. *Pocket Guide to Bach Flower Essences.* Freedom, CA: The Crossing Press, 1997.

Scheffer, Mechthild. *Bach Flower Therapy.* Rochester, VT: Thorsons Publishers, 1987.

Weeks, Nora. *Medical Discoveries of Edward Bach, Physician.* New Canaan, CT: Keats Publishing Co, 1973.

Vibrational Medicine

Gerber, Dr. Richard. *Vibrational Medicine.* Santa Fe, NM: Bear & Company, 1988.

Hunt, Dr. Valerie. *Infinite Mind, the Science of Human Vibrations.* Malibu, CA: Malibu Publishing Co., 1995.

Affirmations

Bristol, Claude. *The Magic of Believing.* Englewood Cliffs, NJ: Prentice-Hall, 1985.

Denning, M. & Phillips, O. *Practical Guide to Creative Visualization.* St. Paul, MN: Llewellyn Publications, 1983.

Dyer, Dr. Wayne. *You'll See It When You Believe It.* New York: William Morrow & Co., 1989.

Ophiel. *The Art & Practice of Getting Material Things Through Creative Visualization.* York Beach, ME: Samuel Weiser, 1984.

Holistic Healing

Borysenko, Dr. Joan. *Minding the Body, Mending the Soul.* New York: Bantam Books, 1988.

Carlson, R. & Shield, B. *Healers on Healing.* Los Angeles: Jeremy P. Tarcher, 1989.

Chopra, Dr. Deepak. *Perfect Health.* New York: Harmony Books, 1990.

Chopra, Dr. Deepak. *Quantum Healing.* New York: Bantam Books, 1989.

Dossey, Dr. Larry. *Recovering the Soul.* New York: Bantam Books, 1989.

Hay, Louise. *You Can Heal Your Life.* Santa Monica, CA: Hay House, 1984.

Krieger, RN, Delores. *Therapeutic Touch.* Englewood Cliffs, NJ: Prentice-Hall, 1979.

Siegel, Dr. Bernie. *Love, Medicine, & Miracles.* New York: Harper & Row, 1986.

Weil, Dr. Andrew. *Health and Healing.* Boston: Houghton Mifflin, 1988.

Spirituality

Borysenko, Dr. Joan. *Fire in the Soul.* New York: Warner Books, 1993.

Foundation of Inner Peace. *A Course in Miracles.* Farmingdale, NY: Coleman Graphics, 1975.

Gawain, Shakti. *Living in the Light.* Mill Valley, CA: Whatever Publishing, 1986.

Hubbard, Barbara Marx. *The Revelation.* Greenbrae, CA: Foundation for Conscious Living, 1993.

Price, John Randolf. *With Wings As Eagles.* Austin, TX: Quartus Books, 1987.

Redfield, James. *The Celestine Prophecy.* New York: Warner Books, 1993.

Roman, Sanaya. *Spiritual Growth.* Tiburon, CA: HJ Kramer, 1989.

Sogyal, Rinpoche. *Tibetan Book of Living & Dying.* San Francisco: HarperSanFrancisco, 1992.

Sugrue, Thomas. *There Is a River.* Virginia Beach, VA: A.R.E. Press, 1945.

Walsch, Neale Donald. *Conversations With God.* Charlottesville, VA: Hampton Roads, 1993.

Zukov, Gary. *Seat of the Soul.* New York: Simon & Schuster, 1989.

Astrology

Hand, Robert. *Planets in Transit.* Rockport, MA: Para Research Publications, 1976.

Lofthus, Myrna. *A Spiritual Approach to Astrology.* New York: Vantage Press, 1980.

Pelletier, Robert. *Planets in Aspect.* Rockport, MA: Para Research Publications, 1975.

Chakras

Judith, Anodea. *Wheels of Life.* St. Paul, MN: Llewellyn Publications, 1987.

Leadbeater, C. W. *The Chakras.* Wheaton, IL: The Theosophical Publishing House, 1974.

Myss, Dr. Caroline. *Anatomy of the Spirit.* New York: Harmony Books, 1996.

Meditation

Leichtman, R. & Japikse, C. Active Meditation. Columbus, OH: Ariel Press, 1982.

Peterson, Richard. *Creative Meditation.* Virginia Beach, VA: A.R.E. Press, 1990.

Tart, Dr. Charles. *Waking Up*. Boston: New Science Library, 1986.

VIDEOS (BACH FLOWER ESSENCES)

The Light That Never Goes Out. The Dr. Edward Bach Center. *Bach Flower Remedies, A Further Understanding*. The Dr. Edward Bach Center.

AUDIO CASSETTES BY RACHELLE HASNAS

• *Affirmations-Enhancing Bach Flower Therapy.....$11.95*
Accompanied by original music, Rachelle offers thirty-eight uplifting affirmations to be used in conjunction with your Bach Flower therapy to enhance flower essence efficacy.

• *To Touch the Light.....$19.95*
This dynamic guided mediation facilitates Chakra alignment and balance, and includes a personal set of seven Chakra Stones to empower your meditation experience.

To order, mail a check or money order in the amount indicated above, plus an additional $3 for shipping and handling to: Rachelle Hasnas, 1063 Tottenham Lane, Virginia Beach, VA 23454

> * The Crossing Press will soon be publishing Rachelle's two new audio cassettes excerpted from her book, *The Essence of Bach Flowers*. Be sure to look for *Traditional Use & Practice of Bach Flowers* and *Transpersonal Use & Practice of Bach Flowers* in the Fall of 1999.

TO PURCHASE BACH FLOWERS

The Bach Flowers are available in most health food stores. If yours does not carry them, they may be ordered directly from the distributor, Nelson Bach, U.S.A, by calling 1-800-319-9151.

Index

BOOKS BY THE CROSSING PRESS

Astrology Alive: *A Guide to Experiential Astrology and the Healing Arts*

By Barbara Schermer

"Schermer brings the astrological chart to life in a way that few other writers have done. It seems destined to become the classic textbook on experiential astrology. It certainly deserves to be."-Howard Sasportas, author of The Twelve Houses

$16.95 • Paper • ISBN 0-89594-873-7

Chakras and Their Archetypes: *Uniting Energy Awareness and Spiritual Growth*

By Ambika Wauters

Linking classic archetypes to the seven chakras in the human energy system can reveal unconscious ways of behaving. Wauters helps us understand where our energy is blocked, which attitudes or emotional issues are responsible, and how to then transcend our limitations.

$16.95 • Paper • ISBN 0-89594-891-5

Color and Crystals: *A Journey Through the Chakras*

By Joy Gardner-Gordon

Information about color, crystals, tones, personality types, and Tarot archetypes that correspond to each chakra. Fully illustrated, indexed and well-organized.

$14.95 • Paper • ISBN 0-89594-258-5

Healing with Flower and Gemstone Essences

By Diane Stein

Instructions for choosing and using flowers and gems are combined with descriptions of their effect on emotional balance. Includes instructions for making flower essences and for matching essences to hara line chakras for maximum benefit.

$14.95 • Paper • ISBN 0-89594-856-7